WITHDRAWN

Springer Series in Cognitive Development

Series Editor
Charles J. Brainerd

Springer Series in Cognitive Development

Series Editor: Charles J. Brainerd

Children's Logical and Mathematical Cognition:
Progress in Cognitive Development Research
Charles J. Brainerd (Ed.)

Verbal Processes in Children:
Progress in Cognitive Development Research
Charles J. Brainerd/Michael Pressley (Eds.)

Adult Cognition:
An Experimental Psychology of Human Aging
Timothy A. Salthouse

Recent Advances in Cognitive Developmental Theory:
Progress in Cognitive Development Research
Charles J. Brainerd (Ed.)

Timothy A. Salthouse

Adult Cognition
An Experimental Psychology of Human Aging

Springer-Verlag
New York   Heidelberg   Berlin

Timothy A. Salthouse
Department of Psychology
University of Missouri-Columbia
Columbia, Missouri 65211 U.S.A.

Series Editor
Charles J. Brainerd
Department of Psychology
University of Western Ontario
London, Ontario
Canada N6A 5C2

With 32 Figures

Library of Congress Cataloging in Publication Data
Salthouse, Timothy A.
  Adult cognition.
  (Springer series in cognitive development)
  Bibliography: p.
  Includes index.
  1. Aging—Psychological aspects. 2. Cognition.
I. Title. II. Series.
BF724.55.A35S24   1982   155.67   82-10584

BF
724.55
A35
S24
1982

Printed in the United States of America

9 8 7 6 5 4 3 2 1

ISBN 0-387-90728-9   Springer-Verlag   New York   Heidelberg   Berlin
ISBN 3-540-90728-9   Springer-Verlag   Berlin   Heidelberg   New York

Series Preface

For some time now, the study of cognitive development has been far and away the most active discipline within developmental psychology. Although there would be much disagreement as to the exact proportion of papers published in developmental journals that could be considered cognitive, 50% seems like a conservative estimate. Hence, a series of scholarly books to be devoted to work in cognitive development is especially appropriate at this time.

The *Springer Series in Cognitive Development* contains two basic types of books, namely, edited collections of original chapters by several authors, and original volumes written by one author or a small group of authors. The flagship for the Springer Series is a serial publication of the "advances" type, carrying the subtitle *Progress in Cognitive Development Research*. Volumes in the *Progress* sequence are strongly thematic, in that each is limited to some well-defined domain of cognitive-developmental research (e.g., logical and mathematical development, semantic development). All *Progress* volumes are edited collections. Editors of such books, upon consultation with the Series Editor, may elect to have their works published either as contributions to the *Progress* sequence or as separate volumes. All books written by one author or a small group of authors will be published as separate volumes within the series.

A fairly broad definition of cognitive development is being used in the selection of books for this series. The classic topics of concept development, children's thinking and reasoning, the development of learning, language development, and memory development will, of course, be included. So, however, will newer areas such as social-cognitive development, educational applications, formal modeling, and philosophical implications of cognitive-developmental theory. Although it is anticipated that most books in the series will be empirical in orientation, theoretical and philosophical works are also welcome. With books of the latter sort, heterogeneity of theoretical perspective is encouraged, and no attempt will be made to foster some specific theoretical perspective at the expense of others (e.g., Piagetian versus behavioral or behavioral versus information processing).

C. J. Brainerd

Preface

This monograph, if successful and not simply ignored, will likely be rather controversial. Perhaps more than in most other fields, researchers in the psychology of aging seem torn in a conflict between scientific and humanistic perspectives. As a consequence, debates concerning the validity and relevance of empirical results often become quite heated and emotional. By attempting to present a strictly scientific viewpoint on the cognitive capabilities of older adults this book will probably strike some humanistically oriented gerontologists and psychologists as being one-sided and overly negativistic. There are also likely to be disagreements within the scientific community concerning interpretations of the research literature since in many cases they contradict commonly accepted (but, I believe, poorly substantiated) beliefs. No guarantee can be provided that my interpretations are any more correct, but the mere existence of rival interpretations should serve to stimulate research that can lead to the resolution of some of these issues.

Adult Cognition will probably also be controversial because serious questions are raised concerning the ultimate usefulness of the research strategy sometimes described as "replicating the *Journal of Experimental Psychology* with an older sample." This approach has obviously led to a vast accumulation of facts about age differences in cognitive processes, but there is reason to be skeptical about whether any genuine advance in knowledge about fundamental aging mechanisms has resulted. Another factor that may contribute to controversy is the rather small size of the monograph. This has imposed limitations on the breadth and depth of coverage, and consequently it is likely that some critics will complain that topic X has been short-changed in its coverage. However, since there would be little agreement as to which topic is topic X, it is impossible to avoid criticism of this type in a relatively short monograph such as this one. And finally, readers used to a traditional organization of topics beginning with simple processes and concluding with complex processes may find the present reductionistic chapter sequence somewhat peculiar. The current organization was adopted because of a philosophical belief that it is useful to understand, or at least describe, what needs to be explained (the complex processes) before examining the mechanisms that might be invoked in the explanations (the simple processes).

While *Adult Cognition* may be controversial for the reasons discussed above, I would like to thank a number of reviewers who did their best to minimize a different type of controversy by pointing out my errors of communication, fact, interpretation, and logic. The students in my Cognitive Psychology course made valuable comments on the entire manuscript, and Chuck Brainerd, Don Kausler, Chuck Krauskopf, Marion Perlmutter, and Ben Somberg offered suggestions on various segments of the book. I would also like to acknowledge my appreciation of the valuable support provided by the staff of the Center for Advanced Study in Behavioral Sciences during my stay there as a Summer Institute Participant in 1980. Special thanks are due those from whom I have learned the most: Jack Botwinick, Bob Gottsdanker, Dick Pew, Ben Somberg, John Stern, Martha Storandt, and Dan Weintraub.

Columbia, Missouri
May, 1982

Timothy A. Salthouse

Contents

Adult Cognition

1. Age and Its Research Significance

Why would anyone want to study the psychology of aging? The popular stereotypes portray the older adult as a fragile and feeble person whose physical and mental capacities are continuously deteriorating. Many people would therefore consider it depressing to focus on the period of decline that seems to characterize the later adult years. Indeed, some cynics might claim that youthful investigators interested in the behavior of older adults have sadistic tendencies, while older investigators are definite masochists.

There are, of course, many reasons besides latent sadistic and masochistic impulses that lead researchers to investigate behavioral aging processes. One reason is simply to explore the validity of the popular myths about aging. It may be that the prevailing stereotypes are inaccurate, out-of-date, or characteristic of only a small proportion of elderly adults. For example, many people automatically associate the later years with a nursing home, and yet some statistics indicate that only about 4% of adults over the age of 65 reside in such institutions (Kastenbaum & Candy, 1973). Similar misleading stereotypes may also exist with respect to the behavioral and intellectual capacities of older adults and thus considerable research is needed to obtain accurate, factual information about this growing segment of the population.

Another major reason for devoting a substantial portion of one's career to the study of adult development is a desire to "cure" or "prevent" the debilities associated with advanced age. Although a skeptic might suspect that investigators pursue this goal for selfish reasons, it is more likely that they are inspired by truly humanitarian concerns since most researchers feel that it is unrealistic to believe that knowledge will accumulate so rapidly that any advances or developments could benefit the present generation. Nonetheless, one can hope that each additional piece of information represents another step towards a "solution" of the "problems" of aging.

A third reason for investigating psychological aging, and the one of primary interest in this book, is a desire to determine the practical importance of aging for functioning in contemporary society. As life expectancy increases and birth rate decreases, it is quite predictable that the average age of the population will increase. Yet, very little is known about the potential effects of this shifting age structure. One of the key issues in assessing the impact of an increasingly older population upon society concerns the ability of older adults to contribute to their community and be self-supporting. The implications for future social policies differ greatly if it is concluded that increased age is characterized by a progressive deterioration of nearly all job-relevant abilities, compared to the conclusion that only sensory acuity and physical strength decline substantially with normal aging. The accurate measurement of changes associated with increased age is therefore essential for rational decision making in the coming years.

In order for this last reason to have much substance in the present context, where much of our discussion will be based on the results of laboratory experiments, it must be demonstrated that the activities in the experimental psychology laboratory are actually relevant to an individual's functioning in the "real world." Such a demonstration has, historically, not been of much interest to experimental psychologists as many have tacitly accepted a distinction between rigor and relevance that is very misleading. Moreover, the artificial nature of the tasks typically employed in psychological experiments has led experimental psychologists to be somewhat defensive about the importance of their work. Even the most seasoned psychological researchers sometimes have doubts about the ultimate applicability of their investigations of the speed with which a person can press a button in response to a light, or the number of repetitions required to learn a list of syllables selected explicitly to be devoid of meaning.

Fortunately for the self-esteem of experimental psychologists, as well as the purposes of the present argument, some limited information is available concerning age differences in professional achievement, industrial job performance, and automobile driving. While this work has not yet been explicitly linked to the results of laboratory investigations, examination of the age trends in these areas is useful in identifying some of the gross phenomena which ultimately must be explained by research investigations in adult cognition. This literature will therefore be briefly described in the following sections to illustrate how the concerns of an experimental psychologist can be relevant to the problems of aging in modern society. Further discussion of the implications of the research findings in cognitive gerontology will be presented in the final chapter.

Professional Achievement

A remarkable assortment of data concerning the years at which individuals in various fields achieve their maximal rates of productivity has been compiled by Lehman (1953). The method was very similar in nearly all of Lehman's analyses. First he located one or more sources that identified major contributions in a particular field. For example, in a scientific discipline he would consult several written histories of that science. Next, the ages of the contributors at the time of the contributions were determined, and tables constructed to indicate the average number of contributions per individual still alive at each age interval. And finally, the values for each age interval were expressed as percentages of the maximum value across all age intervals. It is worth noting that, if anything, this method would tend to underestimate the contributions at young ages because of the inevitable time lag between the initial accomplishment and its later recognition or publication.

Several age functions produced in this manner are illustrated in Figure 1.1 for what Lehman called Scientific fields. Similar functions for Medical fields are portrayed in Figure 1.2. The striking feature of these graphs is that the peak years for productivity occur between age 30 and 40 for nearly all fields, astronomy being the single exception. It is also noteworthy that the rate of achievement drops very rapidly, reaching about 50% of the maximum at around age 50.

One explanation that has been suggested to account for the early peaks and rapid declines of the functions shown in Figures 1.1 and 1.2 is that scientists who make important contributions are likely to be channelled into administrative or supervisory positions, and thus are likely to have less time to make research contributions as they grow older. Lehman offered two rebuttals to this argument. One is that the same general age trends are evident in nonscientific fields such as the creative arts, and in miscellaneous activities such as inventions, chess championships, and geographical discoveries (see Figure 1.3). It seems doubtful that the same trend of advancing eminent individuals out of their original area of expertise would be responsible for the nearly identical functions within each of the fields portrayed in these figures.

Lehman also noted that there were different age functions for the highest quality achievements and for achievements of lesser quality. Figure 1.4 illustrates this difference in the field of psychology. The function labeled "Superior Contributions" represents 85 very distinguished contributions by 50 psychologists, while the function labeled "Lesser Contributions" is based on 4,687 contributions by 339 psychologists. The important point from this figure is that the function for lesser contributions indicates that the individuals do not stop contributing beyond the age of 40, it is just less likely that the contributions beyond those years would be judged as "superior." It still may be that individuals invest less time and effort in projects after the age of 40, but it appears not to be the case that they simply stop making contributions

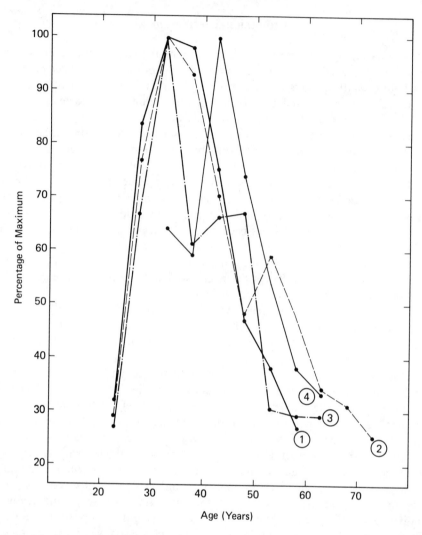

Figure 1.1. Scientific contributions at various ages expressed as a percentage of the maximum number of contributions across all ages. Numbers refer to different scientific areas: 1 = Chemistry; 2 = Mathematics; 3 = Physics; and 4 = Astronomy. Data from Lehman (1953).

because of changing interests or commitments. (See Lehman, 1958a, for a more complete analysis of the difference between superior and lesser contributions in the field of chemistry.)

The most impressive aspect of Lehman's data is that the same general pattern is evident in literally hundreds of analyses across many different areas of endeavor. Regardless of the field, whether it be intellectual, literary, artistic, or athletic, it appears that an individual's most productive period is the

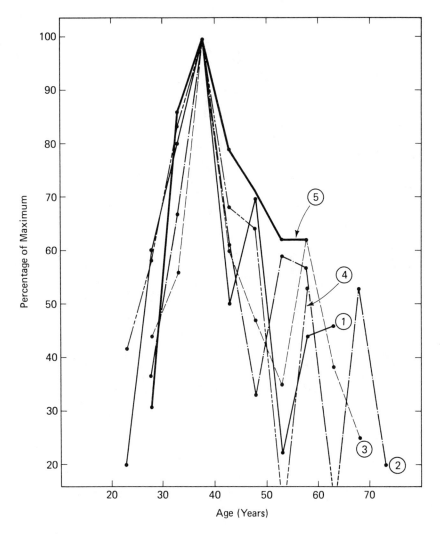

Figure 1.2. Medical contributions at various ages expressed as a percentage of the maximum number of contributions across all ages. Numbers refer to different medical specialities: 1 = Bacteriology; 2 = Physiology; 3 = Pathology; 4 = Anatomy; and 5 = Surgical Technique. Data from Lehman (1953).

decade of the 30s. People beyond the age of 40 still make over one-half of the total contributions in any field, and this figure can be expected to increase as average life span increases, but the greatest rate of achievement seems to occur between the ages of 30 and 39.

An independent analysis of the mean age at which Nobel Prize awardees did the work that led to recognition also found peaks in the late 30s and early 40s (Manniche & Falk, 1957), thus corroborating some of Lehman's results.

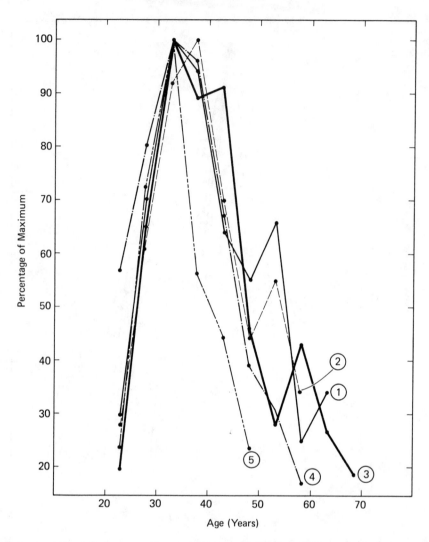

Figure 1.3. Miscellaneous Creative contributions at various ages expressed as a percentage of the maximum number of contributions across all ages. Numbers refer to different fields: 1 = Music, German grand operas; 2 = Art, American sculpture; 3 = Literature, German; 4 = Practical Inventions; and 5 = Chess Championships. Data from Lehman (1953).

In view of the striking implications of these age trends, it is not surprising that many objections have been raised concerning Lehman's methods and analyses. Two of the major criticisms, both initially raised by Dennis (1956, 1958), were anticipated in the 1953 book *Age and Achievement* and subsequently addressed in more detail in separate publications. The first concerned the possibility that anthologists and historians might have had a bias against the recognition of recent contributions such that analyses of at least contem-

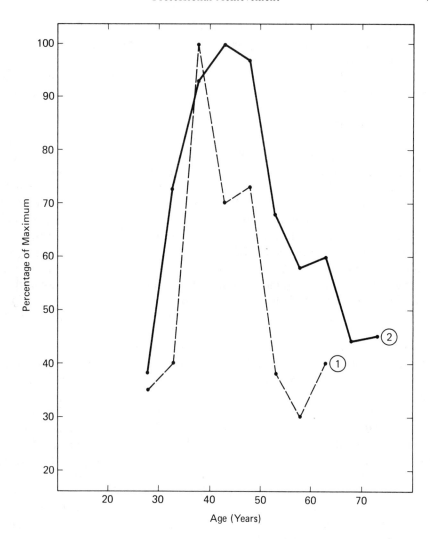

Figure 1.4. Superior and lesser contributions to Psychology at various ages expressed as a percentage of the maximum number of contributions across all ages. The function labeled 1 represents Superior Contributions, and the function labeled 2 Lesser Contributions. Data from Lehman (1953).

porary figures would tend to underestimate productivity at later ages because the contributions were more recent. However, in *Age and Achievement* and in a later article (Lehman, 1962), Lehman reported that very similar age trends were evident in present and past generations of scientists. This tends to disconfirm the recency-bias hypothesis since the same age trends are apparently evident even in much earlier generations of scientists, artists, scholars, etc.

The second criticism dealt with the practice of combining data from persons of different longevities when there were many more people alive to make contributions at younger ages. Separate analyses conducted on individuals of comparable life spans in *Age and Achievement* and in a later article (Lehman, 1958b), revealed nearly the same trends as the other analyses, however, and therefore this hypothesis also seems unlikely (but see Dennis, 1966, for further discussion of this issue).

A more recent criticism was apparently not anticipated by Lehman, but it too seems resolvable with his data. Cole (1979) argued that when the population of potential contributors is expanding and analyses are based on the percentage of individuals making specific contributions, it is more likely that the younger people are making these contributions simply because there are proportionally more of them. This reasoning is compelling if the rate of increase in potential contributors is very large, since even with a constant proportion of quality contributions per age decade, there would be a greater absolute number in the total pool derived from the age group with the largest number of individuals. A limitation of this argument is that one might question whether such a rapid growth in the population of potential contributors occurred in: (a) all fields of endeavor ranging from art to chess to literature to science; (b) all historical times from the 1600s to the present; and (c) a wide variety of countries (Lehman, 1954).

Cole also presented data with a different measure of productivity, and although dismissed as reflecting little or no age trend, they are actually quite consistent with Lehman's results. In analyzing the average number of publications by scientists of different ages, Cole found that the peak productive periods were the ages 40 to 44, and that productivity declined to 77% in the 50s, and 60% in the 60s. The peak years are later and the decline is not as steep as reported in most of Lehman's analyses, but Cole's results are based upon less eminent contributions than those of Lehman and, as discussed earlier, Lehman has found that lesser contributions are maintained better with age than superior contributions. (Thorndike, Bregman, Tilton, & Woodyard, 1928, and Pelz & Andrews, 1966, also found later peaks and flatter decline functions with measures of productivity that are likely to reflect less significant products than those considered by Lehman.)

A longitudinal study of the productivity of mathematicians up to 25 years after receiving their PhD was also reported by Cole (1979), with very little age trend evident throughout the period examined. The contributions were of unknown quality relative to the type chronicled by Lehman, and the age range was only from about 25 to 55, but the absence of a decline would be interesting if extended to a greater age range and confirmed in other fields. At the present time the limited amount of data, relative to the amount indicating a substantial decline, precludes considering these results as anything more than suggestive.

There are undoubtedly many factors responsible for the age trends reported by Lehman, and in fact he mentioned several in discussing his findings. Reduced physical vigor, increased susceptibility to illness, lowered motivation, and less favorable opportunities for concentration were among the alternatives to an age-related reduction in mental ability considered by Lehman. It is almost certainly the case that the progressive changes in lifestyle that occur as one grows older lead to more attention to practical concerns and less freedom from outside distractions. Francis Bacon, the eminent British philospher and politician, noted this tendency nearly 300 years ago in the following statement:

> He that hath both wife and children hath given hostages to the future; for they are impediments to great enterprises, either of virtue or mischief. (1620/1937, p. 21)

Despite the near certainty of a number of factors being involved in the age pattern revealed in Lehman's analyses, the remarkable similarity across the many different fields, and the consistency over a historical period of more than 200 years, suggests that some fundamental characteristic of adult development may be playing a major role. Moreover, it seems likely that the research activities of cognitive psychologists can eventually help to identify this characteristic.

Industrial Work Performance

In view of the extensive age decrements in perceptual and cognitive tasks reported in experimental investigations (to be discussed in later chapters), one might expect to find a strong relationship between chronological age and job performance in many work activities. Indeed, the existence of age differences in nearly all measures of occupational aptitude from the General Aptitude Test Battery (e.g., Fozard & Nuttall, 1971) might be interpreted as indicating that older adults are not suitable for any meaningful employment. However, such a conclusion would obviously be absurd in view of the large numbers of successfully employed older adults. Furthermore, the meager evidence available on industrial job performance does not reveal large age differences (see Arvey & Mussio, 1973; Breen & Spaeth, 1960; Clay, 1956a; King, 1956; Kutscher & Walker, 1960; McFarland & O'Doherty, 1959; Walker, 1964), except in situations where time pressures are present (e.g., DeLaMarre & Shepard, 1958; Mark, 1956, 1957). Workers in their 50s and 60s therefore seem to be just as productive in most jobs as workers in their 20s and 30s.

While the finding that there are little or no age differences in industrial performance might be considered encouraging, one should be cautious about the premature acceptance of this finding. For example, one hypothesis that could account for the lack of an age relationship in industrial tasks is that many older individuals might have left jobs which placed heavy demands upon their declining capacities. In fact, Welford (1958) has claimed that: "The most reliable criterion of difficulty for older people at a job is that substantial numbers leave at a relatively early age" (p. 59). The older workers remaining on a particular job may therefore be highly selected and much less representative of their age group than younger workers.

If this interpretation of the absence of an age difference in measures of industrial productivity is correct, one would expect to find skewed age distributions of workers on jobs with requirements that exceeded the abilities of older workers. That is, there should be relatively fewer older individuals in jobs that are physically or mentally taxing compared to those that make minimal demands on the worker. Evidence for precisely such a skewed age distribution has been reported by Shooter and Belbin in a study described by Welford (1958). These investigators found a striking difference in the age distributions between jobs that involved some type of time stress (e.g., mechanically paced work or piece-rate work) and jobs that did not involve time stress. The most frequent age range in the time-stress jobs was 31–35 for males and 26–30 for females, while the greatest number of workers in jobs without time stress was in the age range 46–50 for both males and females. The identification of time stress as a major factor in the job difficulty of older workers coincides quite well with the literature from laboratory studies indicating that one of the greatest problems of advancing age is a slowing of nearly all aspects of behavior.

A similar confirmation of laboratory findings in engineering and manufacturing industries has been reported by Murrell and his colleagues. Murrell, Griew, and Tucker (1957) and Murrell and Griew (1958) reported consistent age differences in certain jobs in these industries, and Murrell and Tucker (1960) and Griew and Tucker (1958) found that the jobs with age differences could be distinguished by characteristics predictable from laboratory results. For example, Murrell and Tucker identified "vision and perceptual-motor coordination," "short-term memory," and "ability to comprehend and translate" as sources of difficulty in jobs with few older workers, and age-related declines in these abilities have been reported in laboratory studies described by Welford (1958).

Skewed age distributions are also evident in other jobs (e.g., professional athletes, air traffic controllers, etc.), but large-scale meta-analyses combining activities with similar components to rule out idiosyncratic aspects of particular jobs have not yet been conducted. However, a reasonable conclusion based on the existing evidence is that the laboratory discoveries of declining capacities with increased age do have their counterparts in actual work situations. Moreover, it is important to note that the age trends are often apparent as early as the 30s and 40s and do not appear only when the individual is near the age of normal retirement. The "problems of aging" are therefore best conceptualized as beginning at maturity, i.e., between the ages of 25 and 45, rather than at the period conventionally considered to represent the beginning of old age, i.e., age 65.

Before leaving the topic of age and work it is important to correct the impression that may have been conveyed from the preceding discussion that older individuals are invariably a burden, always draining from rather than contributing to the work force. First, it is important to realize that age trends are all based on average results and that the effects of aging are highly individual. Because many older workers may outperform the majority of young workers it is simply not feasible to attempt to predict the performance of a particular individual on the basis of chronological age alone.

And secondly, in many fields on-the-job experience is much more important than perceptual, motor, or cognitive ability, and increased experience is almost inevitably associated with more advanced age. Indeed, several studies have reported little or no age differences in comparisons of experienced workers despite the existence of sizable age differences between inexperienced young and old adults (e.g., Murrell & Edwards, 1963; Murrell & Forsaith, 1960; Murrell & Humphries, 1978; Murrell, Powesland, & Forsaith, 1962). Maher (1955) has reported that older salesmen are rated higher in knowledge of the product than young salesmen, but in other fields it is not yet clear how the greater experience contributes to improved performance. Nonetheless, it seems indisputable that at least in some cases sheer experience can more than compensate for any declining ability associated with increased age.

A third positive aspect of older workers is that the older segment of the working population can make a unique contribution as a direct consequence of their declining capacities. Griew (1959a), Murrell (1962), and Welford (1962) have all noted that in some situations older workers can serve as a test population to determine which aspects of a job or work situation are particularly stressful. The reasoning is that an older worker generally fails at a specific task because the requirements of the task exceed his or her capacities, and when such failure occurs the task is probably close to reaching the limits of the younger worker. Redesign of the job or work environment to fit within the capacities of the older worker will therefore result in an improved work situation for workers of all ages. The following anecdote, attributed to Kleemeier by Griew (1959a), further illustrates this type of unintentional benefit. An enthusiastic, well-meaning geriatric specialist was instructing an architect on the need to design houses for old people with warm and resilient floors when the architect replied: "And for whom, Sir, should I build them cold and hard?" The point, of course, is that any improvement that would benefit the older individual would probably also be appreciated by younger individuals. Older workers are simply in a better position, precisely because of their diminished capacities and abilities, to identify aspects of a job or work situation that can be modified or eliminated.

Automobile Driving

The activity of driving an automobile is very common in modern society and yet the findings from laboratory experiments would lead one to expect that adults would find it increasingly more difficult to drive as they grow older. Specific results will be described in later chapters, but for the present we can summarize the findings by simply stating that sizable age differences have been reported in a variety of abilities presumed to be relevant to driving skill, e.g., vision (both light detection and pattern discrimination), motion judgment, speed of perception, speed of response, and short-term memory. Although these deficiencies might not be evident in normal driving conditions that do not tax a driver to the limit of his or her capacities, when the older person's capacities are exceeded the consequences can be disastrous accidents that are extremely costly both in terms of lives and money.

Statistics on accident rates as a function of the driver's age are confusing as some figures indicate that accident rate decreases continuously from age 25, whereas others indicate that accident rate decreases until about the age of 50 and then begins to increase again. There are probably many reasons for the confusion among the various measures of accident rate, but one of the most important is that individuals of different ages do not drive the same amount and thus the accident rate expressed simply in terms of the number of licensed drivers is misleading (Planek & Fowler, 1971). DeSilva (1938), Marsh (1960), and McFarland, Tune, and Welford (1964) all report that the accident rate expressed in terms of the amount of miles driven begins to increase between the ages of 45 and 60 such that the older driver's accident record is nearly as bad as that of the very young driver. Moreover, even these figures may be underestimates of actual driving ability as it has been found that the type, as well as the amount, of driving differs across age groups (Planek & Fowler, 1971). Older drivers drive less during peak traffic periods and at night when the chances of an accident may be greater. It is also possible that the worst drivers among the older age groups, because of their longer period of exposure, have been removed from the driving population because of an excessive number of violations or involvement in a fatal accident. Taken together, the preceding comments suggest that, in accordance with the expectations from laboratory experiments, the probability of accident involvement increases with increased age beyond the age of approximately 40 or 50.

The types of accidents most prevalent in different age groups are also consistent with speculations from laboratory research. McFarland et al. (1964) report that drivers under the age of 25 are most frequently involved in accidents in which excessive speed, fatigue, or driving on the wrong side of the road were major factors, while drivers 65 and over were more often involved in accidents caused by improper lane changes or turning, failure to yield right-of-way, and ignoring traffic signals. In accord with the laboratory conclusions that age is associated with a widespread behavioral slowing, McFarland et al. (1964), Planek and Fowler (1971), and Planek (1974) have speculated that many of these accidents of elderly drivers are caused by the inability of the older adults to maintain the rapid pace of information processing required by modern driving. Moreover, McFarland, Moseley, and Fisher (1954) point out that the anxiety produced by the older individual's awareness (or fear) of his or her declining abilities may exacerbate the driving impairments.

The problems of the older driver actually extend beyond the driver and his or her passengers as the characteristics of the older driver (e.g., slow speed often impeding the flow of traffic, hesitant actions, improper signalling, etc.) may precipitate accidents in which the older driver does not actually participate. Reduced capacities associated with increasing age may therefore affect everyone, and not merely those currently of advanced age.

An Important Cautionary Note

The preceding three sections have stressed aspects of extralaboratory behavior that exhibit age differences in favor of younger adults. Perhaps even more remarkable in light of the dramatic age differences reported in laboratory studies is the apparent absence of age differences in many activities. Murrell (1965) expressed this view in the following fashion:

> Anyone reading the results of the laboratory experiments could be forgiven for imagining that any person who achieves the age of fifty will have become a slow, forgetful, half-blind, half-deaf, palsied character of little use in industry. In fact, many older men and women hold down jobs with complete satisfaction to their employer. This does not mean that the experimental findings are fallacious. The apparent anomaly seems to derive from the use in the laboratory of subjects who are naive in the practice of the particular faculty which is being tested. (1965, p. 449)

As Murrell notes, the discrepancy between what might be expected on the basis of laboratory results and what is often observed in older individuals is probably attributable to greater experience of older adults relative to young adults. Cognitive psychologists are just beginning to explore the role of experience in skilled activities, but there is already growing awareness that results from unpracticed laboratory tasks may have very limited generalizability to real-world activities. Nowhere is this generalizability problem more severe than in the field of adult development since amount of experience is generally positively correlated with increased age. The challenge for researchers in adult cognition, therefore, is to determine which basic abilities are negatively affected by increasing age, and then to identify the possible compensatory role of experience in allowing maintenance of molar behavior despite declines in component abilities.

In the following chapters we will attempt to identify abilities that are and are not affected by increased age during adulthood, and also strive to specify some of the mechanisms responsible for these changing abilities. Because of the unknown contribution of actual experience, we may not find that all deficits isolated in the laboratory have their counterparts in "real" life. Nevertheless, the laboratory investigations are important if for no other reason than to establish the baseline against which the contributions of experience can be evaluated.

Functional Age

One specific way in which the transition from laboratory to life might be more direct and obvious is in the development of a test battery to assess "functional age." The term "functional age" was apparently first used by McFarland (1953) in a discussion of the need to consider ability to perform the required duties rather than mere chronological age in the evaluation of workers. Although the notion of a functional age test battery has frequently been discussed (e.g., Comfort, 1969; Fozard, 1972; Kaplan, 1951; McFarland, 1973; Nuttall, 1972), only a few large-scale studies have actually been reported. Perhaps the first study of this type was conducted by Glanzer, Glaser, and Richlin (1958) in which 14 intellectual and perceptual tests were administered to over 500 pilots and other aircraft personnel ranging from 21 to 50 years of age. More recently, Dirken (1972) summarized the results from a study of 316 Dutch workers administered a number of physiological and psychological tests, and Heron and Chown (1967) reported the results of a battery of psychological, physical, physiological, and sensory tests given to 540 British adults between the ages of 20 and 79. Szafran (1968) also administered a battery of physiological and psychological tests to several hundred professional pilots. None of the studies carried the project to the stage of examining the relationship between the functional age measures and occupational productivity or performance.

The basic idea behind the functional age concept is to substitute measures indicating the individual's potential for functioning for the variable of chronological age. Chronological age as a classification criterion has been criticized on three grounds. The first, and most important, criticism is that individuals age at different rates and that this individual variation is ignored by the chronological age variable. Since the variability across individuals often increases with age, the chronological age variable may actually be less useful for prediction in the very region of the life span where it is most often relied upon.

The second and third objections concern measurement implications of the chronological age scale, and although seldom explicitly stated, they nonetheless appear to be implicit in many arguments concerning functional age. The second objection is that chronological age, being unidimensional, implies that all aspects of the individual age at the same rate. In other words, knowledge of one's chronological age should be as informative about an individual's decision-making capability as, say, his or her sensory capacities and physical strength. However, evidence of much more rapid age declines in sensory and motor abilities compared to some intellectual and cognitive abilities seems to challenge the validity of this notion.

The third objection is that the interval properties of chronological age lead to a given number of years being assigned the same "meaning" throughout the age scale. That is, the interval between the ages of 43 and 44 is accorded the same status as the interval between the ages of, for example, 0 and 1, even though the latter interval undoubtedly is a period of greater psychological and biological change than the former interval.

The solution to these problems, according to advocates of the functional age notion, is to replace chronological age with an index representing an individual's relative standing on several measures of performance. It is clear that a performance-based index would be more sensitive to individual differences, and thus should lead to greater predictability, than the chronological age measure. Individuals assigned the same functional age would, by definition, possess equivalent skills and abilities even though their chronological ages might vary considerably. Moreover, the units on the functional age scale would be inherently meaningful since they would be expressed in terms of units presumably closely related to performance potential.

The utilization of a relevant functional age assessment would seem to offer definite advantages over the chronological age criterion. Not only could employment and retirement decisions be based on a more rational effective-ability basis, but costly legal suits concerning age discrimination could also be avoided. In this latter connection it is interesting to note Fozard and Popkin's (1978, p. 986) comment that:

> ... experience ... in providing expert testimony regarding abilities and age has resulted in our belief that if a fraction of the money typically spent in court proceedings were spent on applied studies relating measured aptitude to job success, it would in most cases obviate the necessity of the court proceedings in the first place.

Despite the advantages described above, and the general desirability of obtaining an index that has better predictive power than chronological age, functional age measurement will probably not achieve the status that some of its early advocates would have desired. The major problem with the functional age concept is that it, like the chronological age variable it was intended to replace, is a single, unidimensional index that implies related patterns of growth or decline for all abilities and capacities. If mental and physical changes occur independently of one another, no single measure will be very useful for characterizing all aging changes, even if it is based on actual measurement of function. It is also worth noting that to the extent that the various measures contributing to the functional age index are all highly correlated with one another they are redundant, and a single variable might serve as well as a complete battery of variables. This single measure could still be considered an index of functional age, but the available evidence argues against the concept of a universal aging process that produces equivalent rates of change in all abilities.

A related problem with the functional age concept is that different jobs require quite different skills and capacities, and in order for the functional age measurement to be useful the functions must be fairly specific to the job of interest. Indeed, the optimum measure for maximum validity would be actual job performance in order to allow strategies of compensation to be fully employed. However, this implies that no single functional age index can be effective in more than a few related contexts. For example, the criteria used to make a functional age assessment in the field of professional athletics would probably not be relevant in distinguishing among college professors, and supreme court justices would undoubtedly object to being evaluated with the same criteria used to evaluate candidates for womb implants in the role of a surrogate mother. While these examples are somewhat farfetched, the enormous diversity of occupational requirements does make it unlikely that any single measure could ever be of much general value.

A much more reasonable approach advocated by Heron and Chown (1967), although still not free of all of the problems discussed above, is to utilize a functional age profile rather than a single functional age index. An individual's relative position can be determined on a number of variables with reasonably general relevance and "each function can then be considered separately and in relation to the objects for which an assessment of the individual is being made" (Heron & Chown, 1967, p. 141). The use of a multidimensional profile rather than a unidimensional index thus has the advantage of minimizing the tendency to assume that an individual can be accurately described with a single number.

It is in this regard that an analysis of laboratory-based findings concerning age-ability relationships will likely prove useful. Only after the laboratory results have been carefully examined and reliable findings identified can one begin to construct a reasonable functional age battery. Most of the chapters that follow attempt to determine the influence of adult age in a range of abilities; further speculations about the feasibility of a functional age battery are contained in the final chapter.

Summary

Regardless of whether one studies psychological aging for what might be characterized as intellectual, humanitarian, or practical reasons, it is obvious that considerable amounts of accurate information about age differences in behavior are necessary.

A brief examination of age relationships in professional achievement, industrial work performance, and automobile driving revealed that there are sizable age differences in many "real-world" activities. Although most of the research to be discussed throughout this book was conducted in laboratory settings, the evidence suggests that many of the results from laboratory experiments have counterparts in extralaboratory phenomena. In fact, despite the compensatory role of experience, it is possible that a fair percentage of daily activities are affected by the type of ability decrements investigated by cognitive psychologists interested in aging. To take just one example, the laboratory findings indicating that older adults have difficulty with rapidly paced stimulus presentations could be interpreted as suggesting that older individuals are less able to follow and comprehend messages on radio and television. This implication has not yet been directly tested, but Phillips and Sternthal (1977) have used this argument in recommending that advertisers attempting to reach older populations avoid the externally paced electronic media, in favor of such advertising outlets as newspapers and magazines that permit the individual to examine material at one's own pace. While some cognitive psychologists might be reluctant to generalize their results to such "real-world" situations at the present time, it seems indisputable that many of the activities in the cognitive psychology laboratory are relevant to daily experience. It is sometimes difficult to see the overall significance of particular results when one gets immersed in a specific topic, but a global perspective such as that attempted in this chapter usually allows one to determine the pertinence of even the most esoteric research.

Two themes that will persist throughout the book make their first appearance in this chapter. The first is that aging is a very broad phenomenon starting at early maturity rather than at late middle-age as is popularly assumed. Unlike other treatises in adult development, the perspective in this book is that aging is a continuous process that characterizes the ages from about 25 on, and not just the period from age 65 to death. In fact, very little attention will be devoted to ages beyond about 70 to 75 in the subsequent chapters because of the difficulty of studying "normal aging," independent of disease, in very old adults.

The second theme that will be evident in later chapters is that investigation of adult development is plagued by a large number of methodological difficulties and thus an open, flexible approach is required of researchers in this field. Some of these problems were evident in the discussion of research in the areas of work performance and automobile driving, and alternative dependent variables were found to support the hypotheses, despite initially negative evidence. Good research in developmental psychology, even more than is the case in other areas of behavioral science, seems to demand high levels of methodological sophistication and theoretical ingenuity. While not guaranteed to produce sophistication and ingenuity, the following two chapters at least provide a general introduction to the major issues in adult developmental methodology and theorizing.

2. Methodological Issues

It is convenient to introduce the topic of methodology with a concrete, but fictitious, example. We will consider the perspective of a 20-year-old female in the year 1984 who has a desire to find out how she will be different when she is 70 years old, in the year 2034.

One approach the girl might take would be to compare her status to the current status of her grandmother, who is now 70 years old. The grandmother differs from the girl by the appropriate number of years and therefore she might provide a relevant "mirror into the future." However, it is obvious that the grandmother differs from the girl in many respects other than age, and it is possible that one or more of these other differences may distort the "future reflection." For example, the grandmother as a child did not have the opportunity to watch educational television, participate in organized athletic competition, or eat in fast food restaurants, but she could have attended a one-room school, seen the first cross-country airplane flight, or cooked on a wood-burning stove. To the extent that any of these cultural or generational differences influence the variable of interest, this *cross-sectional* comparison of individuals from different age groups at the same point in time may be limited in its ability to predict future age effects. In other words, with this method it is impossible to be certain that the differences between the girl and the grandmother were actually caused by increased age, or were simply the result of different experiences that have accumulated over the years.

A second approach the girl might take to anticipate the effects of aging in her own life is to compare the present status of her grandmother, at age 70, with her grandmother's status at age 20, in the year 1934. Obtaining accurate information over a 50-year span may be quite difficult, but only with such information can the girl examine the changes that occurred in the same person over a period of 50 years. These age changes could then be projected into the girl's own life after an initial adjustment is made for the differences apparent between the grandmother at age 20 and the girl at the present time.

Although the second approach seems to provide a reasonable basis for prediction, this type of *longitudinal* comparison of the same individual over an extended period of time is contaminated by cultural and generational factors in the same manner as the cross-sectional comparison. The problem is that while the grandmother was growing older, from 1934 to 1984, other things in society and culture were also changing that could have contributed to her present status. It is therefore impossible to assume that the changes that occurred to the grandmother between 1934 and 1984 will be identical, or even similar, to the changes that will occur to the girl between 1984 and 2034. Medical advances might lead to the prevention of nearly all diseases, inventions might be introduced to eliminate all manual work, or the fountain of youth might finally be discovered and duplicated for distribution throughout the world. Any of these, or a multitude of other factors, that influence the variable of interest could lead to the changes experienced by the girl between 1984 and 2034 being quite different from the changes experienced by the grandmother between 1934 and 1984.

This brief introduction to the two major research designs in developmental psychology illustrates the general procedures, and some of the difficulties, associated with each design. The remainder of this chapter further examines the major advantages and disadvantages of the traditional cross-sectional and longitudinal developmental research designs, and also a variety of other methodological issues that are necessary to consider when attempting to understand and evaluate human aging research.

Traditional Research Designs

A cross-sectional design is one in which individuals from different ages are compared at the same point in time. This is probably the most popular developmental research design because it is a relatively rapid method for determining age differences. Individuals of different ages are compared at the same point in time, and thus the delay between the formulation of the research question and the availability of the results is determined solely by the time required to obtain measurements from all individuals.

The major disadvantage of the cross-sectional design is that because the individuals of different ages grew up during different periods of time, it is highly likely that they differ in many respects besides age. These generation-specific experiences will be discussed in further detail under the topic of effects of environmental change.

Another problem with the cross-sectional research method is that it is often very difficult to obtain representative samples of individuals from each age group. To the extent that different age samples are not equally representative of their age group it is impossible to separate the effects of age from the effects of representativeness. For example, if a group of college athletes is compared against a group of sedentary 50-year-old office workers on a measure of physical coordination, one should obviously not attribute all differences between the groups to the effects of increased age. The college athletes are undoubtedly more coordinated than the average young adult and thus the sample is not representative of the population of young adults. The office workers may be more representative of their age group, but because they are not highly selected in the same fashion as the young athletes the difference in representativeness contaminates, or is confounded with, the difference in age. The difficulty of obtaining equivalent, unbiased, samples in each age group is a potential problem in nearly all cross-sectional studies.

Longitudinal research designs, in which the same individuals are tested over an extensive period of time, have two major advantages. Clearly the most important is that only with the longitudinal method can individual aging trends be investigated. If it is suspected that individuals differ in their rate or pattern of aging, perhaps because of their genetic background or for other reasons, it is necessary to use a design that allows the same individuals to be followed throughout their lifetime. For many questions, therefore, the longitudinal design may be the only suitable method.

The second advantage often attributed to the longitudinal method is an increased sensitivity for testing age differences because of the greater statistical power when the same individuals are used in all comparison groups. That is, since identical individuals are examined at all ages there is no extraneous individual difference variation to complicate the interpretation of any age differences that might be observed. However, this particular advantage is probably only important when a variable is being investigated that is suspected to have very small age influences.

By far, the greatest drawback of the longitudinal method is the very long time period required to obtain a complete set of observations. The fact that the individuals being investigated have approximately the same life span as the investigator makes it very difficult for a single researcher to carry out longitudinal research. It is more feasible with lower animals that have a short life span, or even with children where the period of interest is only five or ten years, but in the field of human aging the longitudinal method is often impractical because of the tremendous time period involved.

Related to the problem of the extreme time commitments required of longitudinal designs are the disadvantages of expense and inflexibility. Expense is self-explanatory in that some long-term assurance of funds is necessary to carry out an extended longitudinal study. Money for research is often considered difficult to obtain for short-term projects; it is nearly impossible to obtain a guarantee of money for a period extending 20–50 years into the future. Inflexibility is a disadvantage since once the study begins the investigator is obligated to continue with the original procedures even though they may become outmoded or obsolete. That experimental tasks and tests do become obsolete and unpopular is evidenced by the observation that very few of the tasks or tests utilized 50, or even 25, years ago are still employed in contemporary research. As methodology becomes more sophisticated and theoretical perspectives evolve, it is natural to expect that the "tools" of the research psychologist will change. However, it is essential that exactly the same tasks and tests be utilized in all measurement periods in a longitudinal design even if they have been generally abandoned for one reason or another.

Another major problem associated with longitudinal research designs is that it is often difficult to obtain individuals willing to participate in a long-term project, and those who are willing may not be representative of the population of interest. Moreover, even if a representative sample is available initially, some individuals may drop out of the study and those that remain may no longer be representative.

Still another disadvantage of the longitudinal method is the confounding of age and test sophistication, or the amount of specific practice and general familiarity with the experimenter and the testing situation. As the participants in a longitudinal study grow older, they also receive more testing experience and thus any changes observed might be attributable to the effects of prior testing experience rather than to age itself.

As indicated earlier, the longitudinal method also suffers from the problem of separating the effects of age from the effects of societal and cultural change in much the same manner as the cross-sectional method. Any "environmental" events occurring between the first and subsequent measurement periods may have contributed to the differences that were observed, and the basic research design does not allow the sources of the differences to be distinguished.

The major advantages and disadvantages of the two techniques are summarized in Table 2.1. Based on a simple comparison of the number of disadvantages associated with each method, and perhaps more importantly the time advantage of the cross-sectional method, one might expect the cross-sectional method to be more popular with researchers than the longitudinal method. This is indeed the case as a recent survey of publications over a 12-year period which appeared in the *Journal of Gerontology* revealed that studies with cross-sectional designs were reported seven times more frequently than studies with longitudinal designs (Abrahams, Hoyer, Elias, & Bradigan, 1975).

Of much greater significance than their relative frequencies is the comparability of results from the two types of research design. Ideally one would hope that the cross-sectional and longitudinal methods would yield roughly equivalent results. In the event that findings from the two methods are inconsistent, however, explanations would be required to account for the discrepancy. It is therefore useful to reexamine the methods with the goal of identifying characteristics that might account for divergent results being produced by cross-sectional and longitudinal methods.

Table 2.1 Major Advantages and Disadvantages of Traditional Developmental
Research Designs

Design	Advantages	Disadvantages
Cross-Sectional	Quick data collection	Different environmental exposure at various ages Difficulty to obtain equally representative samples in all age groups
Longitudinal	Individual trends can be investigated Increased statistical power	Time-consuming Expensive Methods may become obsolete Participants may not be representative of population Selective attrition may bias results Increased age associated with increased test experience Increased age associated with more recent environmental exposure

One of the clearest differences between the cross-sectional and longitudinal research designs is the amount of testing experience received by the research participants. Participants in a cross-sectional study are tested only once, while those in a longitudinal study are tested at least twice, and often considerably more frequently. If there is any practice or learning effect associated with prior testing, therefore, it would be a factor only in the longitudinal design. It is important to note that the carry-over effects across successive test sessions may be quite subtle, in the form of sensitizing the participant to particular types of information or problems, and need not involve the retention of specific test questions or answers. The repeated testing effects of the longitudinal design may therefore be difficult to detect in many situations, and yet the possibility of an influence of this type cannot be ignored.

Related to the increased sophistication of the participants is the likelihood of a change in the behavior of the experimenter(s) across successive longitudinal testings. It is possible that experimenters change in subtle ways as a consequence of becoming aware of the results from prior testing sessions. If such an experimenter change does occur, it would probably exert a larger effect in longitudinal studies than in cross-sectional studies because the greater interval between testing allows more opportunity for the investigator to become influenced by knowledge of the outcome of prior testing.

A third difference between the two designs is that it is generally more difficult to obtain a representative sample with a longitudinal design. People are frequently willing to participate in a short-term project, where the total time commitment is one or two hours, but are often reluctant to participate in a project extending for years into the future. Moreover, some of the individuals who do agree to participate in the longitudinal study may later drop out of the study for one reason or another such that the final sample is even less representative of the parent population than the initial sample. Different trends with the cross-sectional and longitudinal methods might thus be due to the longitudinal study containing a more highly selected sample of individuals, either initially or after attrition, than the cross-sectional study.

Another factor that might lead to differences between a cross-sectional and a longitudinal study is noncomparable samples in the various age groups in a cross-sectional study. The same individuals serve in all age groups in the longitudinal method, but different individuals are used in each age group in the cross-sectional method. If the participants in the various age groups in the cross-sectional study differ systematically on some variable related to the dependent measure, the results from the cross-sectional study will not be true age differences and hence will not yield the same age trends as a longitudinal study.

The factor most often assumed to be responsible for discrepancies between cross-sectional and longitudinal methods is a differential impact of physical and social environmental change across the two methods. Because the cross-sectional design involves different individuals in the various age groups, all of whom are tested at the same point in time and consequently had different physical and cultural environments during their "critical" childhood and adolescent years, it might be suspected that the effects of changes in society and culture are greater in cross-sectional studies than in longitudinal ones.

Notice, however, that while the longitudinal design controls for environmental effects during the preadult years, it does not control for environmental effects in the pretest years. Consider a longitudinal study initiated in 1935 when all participants were between 15 and 20 years of age. Subsequent tests in 1945, 1955, 1965, and 1975 will be "pure" with respect to the environmental effects occurring in the first 20 years of life since all participants grew up between 1915 and 1940. However these tests are "contaminated" with respect to the environmental effects occurring in the years immediately preceding each test. The test for 15- to 20-year-olds was administered in the depths of the depression, that for the 25- to 30-year-olds was administered in the midst of a world war, etc. This latter environmental effect is controlled by the cross-sectional method since the participants are all tested at the same point in time, but the former, childhood environment effect, is uncontrolled. Discrepancies between the cross-sectional and longitudinal methods might therefore be caused by a differential importance of early, versus recent, environmental change.

This point about the influence of environmental change on longitudinal studies has been made before (e.g., Kuhlen, 1963; Lorge, 1957; Owens, 1966; Schaie, 1972; Wechsler, 1958), but it still has not been widely recognized. It is interesting that the longitudinal method, by controlling childhood environment at the expense of adult environment, implicitly assumes that learning (i.e., the influence of the environment on the individual) is less effective during adulthood than in childhood, a proposition that remains one of the fundamental research questions in adult cognition.

This concludes the discussion of the two traditional developmental research designs. We have seen that although the methods seem simple, the first impression is quite deceptive as each method has a number of severe disadvantages. Because neither method is completely satisfactory it is often suggested that both methods be utilized in order to compare the results obtained with the two types of designs. If there is little or no difference between the results obtained from the two methods, then one would be justified in having great confidence in the validity of the results. On the other hand, if discrepancies are observed then the investigator can examine the procedural differences between the two methods in order to identify the principle factors responsible.

The environmental change factor is of such potential importance in interpreting the results from both cross-sectional and longitudinal studies, as well as in evaluating any disparities between studies utilizing different designs, that it is the subject of extensive discussion in the next section.

Environmental Change Effects

The issue of the role of environmental change factors in adult development can be considered to be another variant of the nature-nurture, heredity-environment controversy that is so pervasive in nearly all areas of psychology. Since the nurturing environment is changing as the hereditary nature of the individual evolves, it is often difficult to determine whether observed age differences are not actually manifestations of environmental changes. The idea that effects of environmental change had to be separated from the effects of maturational change in interpreting age differences has been reintroduced with different terminology a number of times over the past 40 years. Dewey (1939) used the phrase "economic, political and cultural contexts," while Kuhlen (1940) preferred the term "social change," Anastasi (1958) the term "cultural change," and Riegel (1965) "changing times."

The term "cohort effects" was apparently introduced in this context by Schaie (1965), but it has been used primarily as a synonym for generational effects, and thus it tends to minimize the possibility of environmental change influences within a particular cohort or generation. The cohort terminology is also inadequate because a cohort is not by itself an influence, but instead is merely a vehicle by which other factors, such as environmental changes, exert their effects over time. As Horn and Donaldson (1976) state:

> . . .even if all age differences were shown unequivocally to indicate generational differences . . . the differences would be no less real, and there would be no less need to seek understanding of these differences in terms of factors of health and hygiene and experience. . . . (1976, p. 707)

Schaie (1972) did provide one of the best definitions of these nonmaturational effects in referring to them as "a temporally unique generalized input from the environment." One of the advantages of this particular definition is that it is broad enough to encompass aspects of the physical environment such as ambient sound levels, concentration of chemical pollutants in the air and water, climate, etc., as well as such social or cultural environmental factors as education trends, nutrition habits, mass media characteristics, availability of rapid transportation, public attitudes, etc.

The existence of environmental change factors has two important implications for research in adult development. The first is that any developmental trend may be attributed to a maturational (i.e., intrinsic to the individual) effect, or to an environmental (i.e., traceable to factors external to the individual) effect. Unless independent evidence is available to rule out the likelihood of environmental influences, the environmental change factor must be considered as a serious alternative hypothesis to the hypothesis that the source of the observed results is a maturational factor. In other words, because chronological age is not the only variable that is different when making age comparisons, it is impossible to be absolutely certain that the results one observes are caused solely by the factor of increased age. Schaie (1967) was therefore exaggerating only slightly in claiming that "Thus far it seems just as likely that all which has been investigated refers to differences among generations and thus in a changing society to differences which may be as transient as any phase of that society" (p. 131).

The second implication of the existence of environmental change factors is anticipated in the last segment of the above quote by Schaie (1967), and later elaborated by Baltes and Labouvie (1973), Baltes and Schaie (1976), and Willis and Baltes (1980). This concerns the lack of generalizability if all results are specific to a particular physical or cultural context. As Dirken (1972) stated in connection with the influence of environmental change factors in functional age research: "Functional age can be no more than a comparison of age norms at a particular moment in history, in a particular country, for a particular age, and with but a limited period of validity" (p. 14). That is, to the extent that developmental trends are relative to the conditions of the physical and social environment peculiar to a particular time period, it will be impossible to generalize any results to a different environmental context.

Moreover, since the social and physical environment is continuously changing in unpredictable ways, even the abstraction of a "pure age" effect would not allow satisfactory prediction because aging always takes place in some specific environment and the conditions of future environments cannot be accurately anticipated. (It is interesting to note that Conrad, 1930, recognized this problem many years ago in a discussion of the difficulty of evaluating the future impact on specific test performance of new inventions such as the radio!)

This argument, that the existence of substantial environmental change effects may restrict one's conclusions to a specific temporal-cultural context, seems to deny the possibility of ever attaining a real science of adult development. If all of our facts have to be revalidated after every change in the physical or social environment, there would be little hope of ever discovering truly general laws of human aging.

Fortunately we will see that the data indicate that this pessimism is not fully justified, at least with respect to the type of variables of primary interest to cognitive psychologists. It is undoubtedly the case that when environmental change does have an effect, its magnitude varies substantially across dependent variables. For instance, Botwinick (1978) noted that "social" variables like religious beliefs might be expected to be much more sensitive to cultural change than would "biological" variables such as reaction time. Most cognitive psychologists at the current time probably adhere to such an assumption and, rightly or wrongly, tend to minimize the role of environmental change factors in the interpretation of their results.

A Research Design Sensitive to Environmental Change

A research design that would allow independent assessment of the effects of environmental change was first discussed by Anastasi (1958), and later elaborated by Riegel (1965), Schaie (1965), and Baltes (1968). The basic idea is to combine the data from two (or more) cross-sectional or longitudinal studies conducted at different points in time. For example, let us assume that a cross-sectional study was conducted in 1930 with groups of 20-year-olds and 70-year-olds, and that another identical study was conducted in 1980 with new samples of 20-year-olds and 70-year-olds. (The 70-year-olds in 1980 need not be the same individuals who were the 20-year-olds in 1930; this is the distinguishing characteristic of independent-sample or repeated-sample versions of this design.) Comparisons in either 1930 or 1980 between the 70-year-olds and the 20-year-olds are, as was discussed earlier, confounded by a mixture of maturational changes and environmental changes. However, an estimate of the magnitude of environmental influences can be obtained by comparing individuals of the same age tested at different points in time. For example, the difference between the 20-year-olds tested in 1930 and the 20-year-olds tested in 1980 is, if the procedures and measurement methods were identical, an estimate of the effect of general environmental change during the

Table 2.2 Removing the Effects of Environmental Change

	Year	
	1930	1980
	A (20-year-olds)	C (20-year-olds)
	B (70-year-olds)	D (70-year-olds)

Possible Influences

Comparisons	Maturation	Environmental Change
B versus A	Yes	Yes
D versus C	Yes	Yes
C versus A	No	Yes
D versus B	No	Yes
C versus B	Yes	Yes
D versus A	Yes	Yes

50-year period between 1930 and 1980. (See Table 2.2 for a summary of this reasoning.)

If there is no difference between the measurements of individuals of the same age at different periods of time one can assume that changes in the environment had little or no influence on that particular dependent variable. Under these circumstances the investigator is probably justified in interpreting differences between age groups as being primarily determined by maturational factors. That is, in the terminology of Table 2.2, both cross-sectional (e.g., D vs. C) and longitudinal (e.g., D vs. A) comparisons provide accurate estimates of maturational effects if the time-lag difference (e.g., C vs. A) is very small.

Interpretations are considerably more difficult if there is a difference as a function of time of measurement in individuals of the same age. This outcome would indicate that environmental change factors are important in influencing the dependent variable, and therefore one could not attribute differences between age groups solely to maturational processes. An estimate of the maturational contribution might still be possible when environmental effects cannot be ignored by adhering to the following procedure. First, the magnitude of the environmental change effect for the period of interest is obtained by comparing the measurements of one age group at two different times, in the manner described above. Next, the combined maturation-plus-environment effect is determined by contrasting the age groups at the most recent measurement period. That is, the difference between 70-year-olds and 20-year-olds in 1980 is assumed to be caused by both maturational and environmental factors. Finally, the environmental change effect can be subtracted from the maturation-plus-environment effect to obtain an estimate of only the maturation contribution.

Even this rather complicated approach has at least two important limitations. The first is that if the environmental factors differentially influence some age groups more than others environmental effects will have to be estimated separately for each age group that is being evaluated. Thus, the difference between 20-year-olds in 1980 and 20-year-olds in 1930 would estimate the impact of environmental change in educational practices and other factors influencing the first 20 years of life, but it would not provide comparable information about changes in health practices, social services, or attitudes that primarily affect older individuals. In order to obtain an estimate of this type of age-specific environmental change it is necessary to compare 70-year-olds in 1980 with 70-year-olds in 1930. The problem then arises as to which environmental change estimate is to be subtracted to obtain a pure measure of maturational effects. Subtracting the 20-year-old estimate essentially equates the 20-year-olds and the 70-year-olds at age 20, but all environmental changes that selectively influence the ages between 20 and 70 are ignored. Subtracting the 70-year-old estimate seems more appropriate because it takes into account the cumulative environmental change throughout the individual's life, but it fails to provide any period in which the age groups being compared could be considered equivalent.

A second limitation of this approach to estimating the maturational component is that because the environmental effects are always changing, the generalized environmental input that is subtracted from the observed differences must correspond exactly to the time period separating the age groups. In other words, it is feasible to subtract the 1930–1980 environmental change effect from the 1980 comparison of 20-year-olds and 70-year-olds because the 50 years between 1930 and 1980 represent the actual years that the 70-year-olds were in the environment between the ages of 20 and 70. However, it is not legitimate to subtract the 1930–1980 environmental change effect from the 1930 comparison of 20-year-olds and 70-year-olds unless one assumes, in direct contradiction to the "temporally unique" premise of the environmental change argument, that the period from 1880 to 1930 was essentially equivalent to the period from 1930 to 1980.

The estimation of the contribution of environmental change is therefore hampered by the fact that the change is unsystematic and cannot be easily predicted. Indeed, Schaie (e.g., Schaie & Labouvie-Vief, 1974; Schaie, Labouvie, & Buech, 1973; Schaie & Strother, 1968a) has reported that the same time period may exert a positive effect on some variables (e.g., vocabulary and general information scores), and a negative effect on others (e.g., perceptual-motor speed). Another problem with estimating the magnitude of the environmental change effect is in obtaining comparable intervals of time for the environmental and maturational estimation periods. As Botwinick and Arenberg (1976) and Adam (1977) have recently pointed out, the estimates may be misleading if, for example, a 50-year maturational difference is evaluated against a 7-year difference attributable to environmental change.

The preceding discussion indicates that the multiple or sequential (multiple cross-sectional) design is an improvement over traditional cross-sectional or longitudinal designs in allowing more precise conclusions if: (a) there are no differences as a function of time of measurement, indicating that the environmental change contribution is negligible; or (b) very strong assumptions are made concerning the systematic nature of environmental changes so that the environmental factor can be subtracted out of the observed differences to produce a net maturational effect.

It should perhaps be noted that in Schaie's (1965) description of this procedure, two additional research designs were also proposed to obtain separate estimates of the effects of what he referred to as cohort and time-of-measurement. It has since been convincingly argued (e.g., Adam, 1978; Baltes, 1968; Buss, 1973; 1979; Horn & Donaldson, 1976; Schaie & Baltes, 1975) that time-of-measurement and cohort cannot be empirically distinguished and hence that Schaie's initial formulation was apparently unnecessarily complicated. The sequential cross-sectional design described above therefore seems to represent the current consensus on the best manner of dealing with environmental change effects in a developmental study.

Although this combined design may be the best available method for separating maturational and environmental determinants, it is not without severe flaws. In fact, in combining features of the cross-sectional and longitudinal designs it might appear that the sequential cross-sectional design has retained nearly all of the disadvantages inherent in the original designs. As in the cross-sectional design, the validity of any conclusions is heavily dependent upon the various samples being equally representative of their parent populations, i.e., that age group at that particular time. In commmon with the longitudinal design are the disadvantages of the long time period required before complete observations are available, the expense associated with long-term projects, and the problem of procedures becoming outmoded or obsolete.

Two variants of the design discussed above can occasionally be employed to overcome some of these disadvantages. One alternative approach is to compare cross-sectional samples at the same point in time from two or more populations that are known to differ in important cultural characteristics. For example, young and elderly adults in an urban, Western society could be compared with young and elderly adults in a rural, undeveloped society. If the differences between young and old adults are fairly similar in the two societies, one could infer that the environmental factor probably does not influence the developmental differences for that particular dependent variable. Unfortunately, no simple interpretation is possible if the age trends are different in the two societies.

The second alternative is to select a population whose environment has not changed significantly for an extended period of time. This is probably feasible only with very primitive societies or with lower animals, but the results from a cross-sectional study with such a population could be important in providing an accurate estimate of maturational effects uncontaminated by differential environmental experiences.

To many researchers the debate concerning the relative importance of maturational and environmental factors is a rather esoteric and fruitless controversy. One indication of this attitude is the nearly exclusive use in the contemporary research literature of the phrase "age differences" rather than "age changes." Use of the former term connotes a recognition that nonmaturational factors may be contributing to the results one observes, but with a realization that the phenomena still require some type of explanation.

Internal and External Validity

Perhaps even more than in almost all other areas of science, investigators in adult development must be sensitive to issues of internal and external validity in designing and interpreting research. Internal validity refers to the degree to which differences in the dependent variable may be attributable to the independent variables of interest, rather than to irrelevant, extraneous variables. High internal validity is therefore essential in order to make meaningful statements about the results of any research project. External validity refers to the degree of generalizability of the specific sample of conditions, measures, and participants to the populations of interest. If the results of an investigation are applicable only at a unique time or place, or only with certain dependent variables, or only with a particular set of people, they will not be generalizable and hence will have little or no value beyond the specific situation in which the data were collected.

Many of the factors discussed in the preceding sections primarily affect internal validity in that they tend to obscure the relationship between the chronological age variable and the dependent variable of interest. However, both internal and external validity could be influenced by the environmental change factor since it could distort the relationship between age and the dependent variable, and also restrict any generalizations to the particular environmental context in which the observations were made. A number of other factors of special significance to developmental researchers can also affect both internal and external validity and thus they too must be considered when designing, interpreting, or evaluating developmental research.

It is well accepted that the best assurance of external validity is random selection of research participants, and that the best assurance of internal validity is random assignment of participants to groups or conditions. Unfortunately, neither of these techniques is possible for investigators in adult development. Individuals might be selected randomly from a population, but many will refuse to participate in a research project and the ones that do participate may no longer constitute a random sample. And while it might be possible for an investigator to induce rapid aging in a young individual by chemical or electrical stimulation, it is currently beyond the powers of even our most capable investigators to restore the youth of an older individual so that participants could be assigned to age groups on a random basis. Researchers concerned with processes of aging must therefore rely on compromise techniques in the attempt to maximize internal and external validity.

Problems with Selection of Research Participants

The selection or procurement of individuals to participate in a developmental research study involves a number of problems. First, because individuals cannot be forced to participate in a project, there may be some selection bias in that the volunteers who do participate may not be representative of the total population. Any selection bias of this type may weaken the external validity of the study.

Second, since volunteers are needed, investigators often attempt to recruit participants from groups or institutions where there is the greatest likelihood of obtaining volunteers. If the members of these groups or institutions are not representative of the general population, results cannot be widely generalized and thus the external validity is further reduced. Internal validity would also be jeopardized if the various age samples are not obtained from the same sources. For example, if young adults are recruited from college classrooms while older adults are recruited from senior citizen clubs or retirement organizations, the two age groups will differ in many ways other than age. If any of these other factors is related to the measure of interest the age relationship will be impossible to interpret because of low internal validity.

A third problem related to the previous one concerns the use of "subject pools" with one or more age groups. It has long been common practice in colleges and universities to encourage students to participate in research projects for scientific, educational, monetary, or other reasons. In certain research centers, it is also becoming popular to establish such "subject pools" with groups of middle-aged and elderly individuals. The problem with this practice is that once an individual participates in a single project he or she is no longer as representative of the population as before the participation. In many cases the contamination caused by prior participation will be very slight because quite different phenomena are being investigated in each participation. Strictly speaking, however, external validity is reduced by utilizing individuals who are known to have participated in one or more prior studies. Internal validity could also be affected if one age group has received more prior participation than another. This is often the case when college students serving in several experiments as a course requirement are compared against typical (i.e., first-time participant) older adults, or when older participants in a longitudinal study are contrasted with naive young individuals.

In light of the difficulties associated with obtaining adequate samples of individuals in different age ranges it is useful to list some of the successful procurement techniques employed by earlier investigators. Certainly the most common means of obtaining adult research volunteers has been to make contact with an existing organization such as a church, social group, or club, and attempt to enlist the cooperation of the leaders. Some of the loyalty and cooperative spirit associated with the group might then generalize to the experimental situation. Moreover, when research funds are available for compensating participants the groups can encourage research participation as a fund-raising activity for the organization. The investigator should be aware, however, of the possibility that individuals who join groups may be positively selected and not representative of the general population.

Other recruitment strategies have been to request participation of members of a family medical health plan (e.g., Schaie, 1958), borrowers from the Farm Security Administration (e.g., Heston & Cannell, 1941), parents of elementary school or college students (e.g., Christian & Paterson, 1936; Willoughby, 1927), individuals seeking aptitude information from a commercial career counseling center (e.g., Trembly & O'Connor, 1966), or prison inmates (e.g., Corsini & Fassett, 1953; Demming & Pressey, 1957; Horn & Cattell, 1966, 1967; Horn, Donaldson, & Engstrom, 1981; Mursell, 1929; Thorndike et al., 1928). Weisenburg, Roe, and McBride (1936) obtained participants from a hospital population, arguing that in very few situations can one find such a wide age range of individuals with relatively large amounts of free time. Thorndike and Gallup (1944) were able to obtain an extremely representative sample by incorporating their research questions into a national opinion poll. A similar broad sample, although of uncertain representativeness, was obtained by Broadbent and Gregory (1965) by using public television for the presentation of their test material and having participants mail in their responses.

One of the most unusual recruitment techniques was employed by Jones, Conrad, and Horn (1928) who offered free movies to potential participants in rural New England communities. The movies were thought to create an atmosphere of goodwill and inspire a friendly cooperative attitude among the participants.

The earliest recruitment technique, and still one with great potential, was Galton's (1885) testing of the visitors to an International Health Exhibition. Galton was actually able to charge his participants for the opportunity to be measured and evaluated, and while this might not work in current times, it should still be possible to obtain large samples of individuals of a variety of ages by recruiting from visitors to county and state fairs, conventions, or large sporting events. Chapanis (1950) used this technique to collect visual sensitivity data on 574 visitors to the Baltimore Sesquicentennial Exhibition.

Attempts to Artificially "Equate" Age Groups

The difficulty of obtaining comparable groups of individuals in the various age categories in a developmental study has already been discussed, and it may very well be impossible to find individuals who differ from one another only on the basis of chronological age. Techniques of matching individuals in the various groups on the basis of some criterion variable, or attempting post hoc statistical equating procedures such as the analysis of covariance, are frequently used to achieve equivalent groups. However, both techniques have many problems of their own. One of the most serious of these problems is that in our present state of knowledge it is nearly impossible to specify which variables are relevant to other variables, and thus there is little justification for selecting a particular variable as the matching or criterion variable.

Even after a relevant variable has been selected, the problems are still not solved as it is possible that matching may actually reduce both external and internal validity. For example, many aging studies have been reported in which the investigator matched young and old research participants on the basis of the number of years of education to avoid differential influence of this factor on the dependent variable. However, since educational trends have changed dramatically over the last 50–100 years, individuals with the same level of education are probably not equally representative of their age groups. An older adult with a college education is likely to have come from a wealthier, more highly educated family than a young college graduate. The technique of matching may therefore create differential representativeness in the two age groups and impair both external validity, by making each sample less representative of its parent population, and internal validity, by introducing a difference in representativeness that is confounded with the difference in age. With some matching variables, e.g., amount of gray hair or smoothness of skin, the process of matching might even result in the elimination of the age effect because the matching variable is inherently associated with a basic aging process.

There is also a statistical problem associated with the matching procedure. If the matching variable is not highly correlated with the dependent variable and individuals are selected from the extremes of each age group in order to produce matched samples, the results may be susceptible to a statistical regression artifact. This occurs because there is some error associated with the initial assignment of individuals, and since they were selected from the extremes of the distribution the error is most likely in the direction away from the mean of the distribution. A second measurement of the matching variable, or of the weakly correlated dependent variable, is therefore likely to fall closer to the mean of its distribution than the original measurement.

An example will help clarify this issue. Let us assume that an investigator matches young and old individuals on the basis of quickness of finger reaction time, and then compares the two groups on a measure of memory ability. It is probable that only the slowest of the tested young participants and the fastest of the tested old participants were used in the matched sample because it is generally reported that reaction time slows with increased age. Now if the memory measure is only slightly correlated with the reaction time measure, it is likely that the participants will not be perfectly classified with respect to memory ability. Moreover, the expected effect of this error is to make subsequent measurements less extreme than the initial measurement. This will cause the participants to be closer to the average of their respective distributions on the memory measure than they were on the reaction time measure. That is, regression to the mean will lead to the young adults performing higher than one might expect, and to the older adults performing lower than one might expect, with the memory variable. The consequence of matching in this case, therefore, might be to produce artificially large age differences even if none really existed.

Health

Even with the best methodology it may be impossible to distinguish the effects of some factors from the effects of normal aging. Health is one such factor in that it is sometimes claimed that many of the effects attributed to increased age are really caused by general or specific deterioration of health. That health problems typically increase with increased age is indisputable. One manifestation of these health problems, the percentage of people reporting various types of health-related activity limitation, is illustrated in Table 2.3. The increase in activity limitation parallels the rise in behavioral impairments reported in a variety of experimental tasks, and thus is consistent with the possibility that poor health and not "normal aging" might be responsible for many of the differences observed in aging studies.

Many investigators attempt to control for the influence of health factors by screening research participants for specific illnesses or cardiovascular problems. For example, a health questionnaire might be administered and only those individuals relatively free of serious health problems might be included in the data analyses. While generally commendable, two limitations of this procedure should be pointed out. First, if the incidence of health problems tends to increase with age, then selecting only those individuals without health problems results in a very biased sample of older adults. To take an extreme example, assume that only 5% of the people between the ages of 65 and 70 are

Table 2.3 Percentage of Health-Related Activity Limitations by Age

Age Range	Limited, But Not in Major Activity	Limited in Amount or Kind of Major Activity	Unable to Carry on Major Activity
17-44	3.2	4.2	1.0
45-64	5.0	12.4	6.1
65+	6.7	21.7	16.6

Note. 1978 data from Table 24 (p. 159) in *Health United States 1980.* U.S. Department of Health and Human Services, Hyattsville, Md., 1980.

completely free of serious health problems (undoubtedly a gross exaggeration). If a researcher restricts his or her investigations to completely healthy older adults, generalizations might be possible only for 5% of the population in that age range.

A second related problem concerns the extent to which aging is itself a disease. There is still considerable controversy among biologists and physiologists about whether normal aging should be characterized as a breakdown in immunities to disease, or even a disease itself. If normal aging is in fact a disease, then attempting to control for health factors may actually result in the elimination of the primary aging effect.

These considerations are mentioned not to dissuade researchers from attempting to disentangle illness from aging, but rather to point out that there is no simple solution to this problem. Certain obvious health problems can be controlled with careful selection of participants, but it may be years before a definitive conclusion can be reached regarding the status of aging as a disease. Health factors therefore cannot be ignored, although it should be pointed out that most of the research to be discussed in this book has involved noninstitutionalized older populations who report themselves to be in moderate to good health.

Concluding with an Optimistic Perspective

Some readers might feel that the discussion in this chapter has been unduly pessimistic about the problems of conducting aging research. This opinion is obviously not shared by the author as it is claimed that methodological issues, no matter how subtle they might appear, are fundamental in the evaluation of all knowledge. Moreover, only a small proportion of the methodological issues relevant to developmental research have even been discussed here. For example, no mention has been made of the difficulty of obtaining objective information about the most basic variable in developmental research—an individual's age. Most investigators rely on self-reports for chronological age classification, but it is possible that these reports are systematically distorted among individuals in certain age groups. (It is interesting that apparently only two studies—Garfield & Blek, 1952, and Garrison, 1930—have even attempted to address this problem.)

Despite the enormous number of methodological concerns, and the apparent impossibility of satisfactorily addressing all of them in a single study, there are several reasons why we should not become discouraged and abandon our attempts to investigate developmental phenomena. First, it is likely that several of the issues discussed earlier will be found to have little or no impact on many variables. It has already been mentioned that many cognitive psychologists implicitly assume that the measures of interest to them are only minimally affected by social or cultural change. Once this assumption is explicitly tested and confirmed (perhaps by demonstrating that most or all of the observed age differences are determined by experimentally manipulable variables), many of the concerns related to environmental change factors might safely be ignored. Until the rival hypotheses to the maturational explanation have been thoroughly investigated, however, the cautious approach outlined in the preceding pages seems justified.

A second reason for not becoming excessively pessimistic about the prospects of a science of adult development is that no area of science has an abundance of critical studies which unequivocally resolve an issue to the complete satisfaction of everyone. Nearly all research reports have certain flaws or weaknesses that limit the conclusions that can be drawn. Most results must therefore be considered suggestive rather than definitive. This situation is simply magnified in developmental research because of the enormous number of variables which some researchers might consider important. The solution to this problem is to base conclusions on a number of independent research studies, each employing slightly different procedures and measures. With variation in procedures different studies will likely have different flaws, but if consistent age trends are still obtained one can conclude that the specific methodological characteristics are relatively unimportant. It is also a good idea to utilize larger sample sizes than the 10–20 individuals per age group typically used at the current time. This practice will lead to more stable estimates of the quantitative relationship between age and performance, instead of merely demonstrating that a statistically significant difference exists between various age groups.

The viewpoint that scientific confidence should accrue to conclusions based on findings from a number of different studies rather than a single "perfect" study has also been expressed by Welford (1957):

> ... it seems ... clear that no one way of studying ageing is wholly free from methodological objections and that we can thus seldom, if ever, draw certain conclusions from a single experiment or industrial study. In view of this it appears wiser to carry out several small-scale studies using different methods rather than concentrate the whole research on a few large-scale investigations. (p. 168)

This approach of emphasizing conclusions based on aggregate results rather than the findings of a single experiment will be followed throughout this book. Such a strategy may be excessively conservative and could result in the neglect of potentially important discoveries, but until they have been verified in one or more additional contexts there is the risk that the results are not generalizable because of the kinds of methodological issues discussed in this chapter.

Summary

The purpose of the present chapter was to examine some of the methodological issues that complicate the interpretation of research in adult development. We noted that neither the traditional cross-sectional or longitudinal research design is very satisfactory for investigating the effects of aging, and that even a more complicated design incorporating features of both designs is not without severe problems. The enormous difficulty of attempting to achieve maximum internal and external validity in studies of adult development was also discussed. It was argued that the results of single studies in adult development should merely be considered suggestive, and that definite conclusions should only be drawn when similar results are obtained from several different studies each employing different individuals, procedures, and dependent measures.

3. Theoretical Considerations

It is generally recognized that the two primary functions of a scientific theory are to provide a framework for organizing and integrating the existing results, and to suggest directions for future research by specifying important issues for investigation. Both organization and direction seem to be lacking in the current literature on adult cognition and thus there is evidently a great need for theoretical development in this area. Charles (1973), Birren and Renner (1977), and Birren, Woods, and Williams (1980) have also argued that more theories are needed because the predominantly problem- and data-oriented nature of contemporary adult developmental psychology has resulted in a loosely related collection of concepts and hypotheses in which experimentation is often limited to narrow, and frequently trivial, problems.

Although it might be considered premature because very few explicit theories have yet been formulated, an attempt will be made throughout this book to examine theoretical perspectives in adult cognitive psychology. There are several advantages to conducting such a theoretical analysis at the current time. One of these involves determining whether any of the existing theories can serve to organize a substantial amount of data, or whether completely new theories will have to be developed. Facts are accumulating at a rapidly accelerating pace in the field of adult cognition, and unless theoretical frameworks are available to organize these facts they may become overwhelming and consequently be ignored because they are impossible to assimilate.

A second advantage of examining theoretical models of aging is to determine the practical significance of the current research on the psychology of aging. The research literature can be of very little use unless theoretical frameworks are available to allow predictions which apply to extralaboratory contexts. A few limited predictions might be possible on the basis of results from individual studies, but predictions of a more general nature require the systematic, integrated knowledge provided by theories. Moreover, the inter-action between theory and application is actually two-sided since the validity of the theory can be assessed by examining the accuracy of predictions in real-world environments.

The third advantage of attempting a theoretical examination at the present time is to identify major issues for future research. It is probable that many current topics of investigation are primarily of historical significance, without any clear practical or theoretical importance. Unless theories are available to serve as guiding frameworks, research questions may be dictated by conven-ience and personal interest rather than true importance. This is unfortunate because the results of studies directed at such questions are unlikely to make a substantial contribution to knowledge.

A fourth and final reason for examining theoretical issues at this time is the desire to bring the debate concerning the nature of age differences in cognition into the scientific realm, and out of the arena of polemics. Many contemporary researchers become very emotional in discussing the interpre-tations and implications of aging research, apparently because of conflicts in beliefs that are seldom justified on scientific grounds. It is probably also true that many important editorial decisions in journals and merit ratings in funding agencies have been influenced by the implicit assumptions held by the reviewers about the underlying basis for the age differences that are frequently observed in scientific research. Some of the polarization and misunderstanding that currently characterize the field of adult cognition might be minimized by simply making the theoretical issues explicit, and beginning to examine the scientific evidence relevant to each. Only by relying on scientific observation and rational debate can one hope to avoid the fruitless controversy reflected by such emotion-laden and often meaningless comments as "inappropriate interpretation," "negative (or positive) bias," or "misdirected research em-phasis." Each of these and other similar phrases clearly implies a particular theoretical perspective, and a first step in evaluating the adequacy of a perspective is to make the assumptions overt and explicit.

Difficulties of Theorizing in Adult Development

Theorists in the field of aging are confronted with a unique problem not faced by theorists in other areas. Most theorists need to account for some limited amount of psychological activity, but theories in aging are required to explain the *change* in activity, and not just the activity itself. Since the necessity of explaining how a process changes presumably demands a more detailed knowledge than that required for the initial explanation of the process, it follows that theoreticians in adult development often have a more difficult task than their counterparts in other disciplines.

Some researchers in aging have attempted to avoid this difficulty by utilizing existing theories in a parent or related discipline to serve as the framework for interpreting results in aging studies. For example, a researcher interested in perception and aging might adopt one of the theoretical perspectives from contemporary perception research to serve as the framework for guiding and interpreting investigations of age differences in perception. There are both benefits and costs associated with this "borrowing from the mainstream" strategy. Of course the obvious benefit is that the investigator is relieved of the necessity of formulating an original theory, and can simply incorporate the theoretical concepts already developed in his or her "explanations" of aging phenomena. Moreover, in many cases theories borrowed in this manner will be well-supported with a single population of individuals (e.g., young adults), and thus the concepts are already known to have a certain amount of experimental validity.

This advantage is by no means trivial, and some researchers have even gone so far as to argue that:

> a concept or problem . . . should *not* be studied in older adults until a sufficiently verified theory has been developed that accounts for the young adults' performance. (Giambra & Arenberg, 1980, p. 257)

Such a position is understandable if one adheres to the perspective, described by these authors, that the psychology of aging is the "back wheel" to the "front wheel" of mainstream psychology, and as in a bicycle, the back wheel must always follow the front wheel. There is clearly some validity to this viewpoint, but it should not be blindly accepted without consideration of the disadvantages.

Two of the disadvantages or costs attached to this strategy of borrowing theories from other areas to serve as theories of aging are that the original theories may not be relevant for developmental issues, and that the theoretical interpretations that eventually result from this approach are often more analogous to descriptions than explanations. With respect to the first point, it is actually rather presumptuous to assume that merely because a theory has been found to provide a satisfactory description of a particular type of behavior in one group of individuals that it will also serve to describe the manner in which that behavior differs across two or more groups of individuals. In other words, the simple existence of theoretical concepts offers absolutely no assurance that an explanation can be provided for the processes of change, or the dimensions of difference. The change might be qualitative, in the form of a completely different structural organization of processes, rather than quantitative, in the form of reduced efficiency in one of the postulated processes. In a related vein, Baltes and Willis (1977) have pointed out that unless the theory attempts

> . . . to explicate a process of development, then aging subjects continue to be experimental constants leading to parametric variation of principles formulated within a framework of general experimental psychology rather than to a psychology of aging. (p. 144)

Such imported theories should thus be used primarily as a source of hypotheses until sufficient evidence is available within the aging literature to justify their role in actual explanations of aging phenomena.

Theories introduced into the field of aging from other fields are also limited in that the goal with such theories is generally to localize the effects of aging in a specific theoretical structure or process, but no explanation is offered to account for why, or how, age influences that particular structure or process. In a sense, therefore, the researcher employing this strategy has only described an age difference (although generally with more precision than before). Unless some explanation is then furnished to specify why that particular process or structure was affected by age and not some other, and to describe the nature of the developmental changes within the relevant component, the outcome of this strategy is just more description and not actual explanation.

As an example, it has occasionally been claimed that the age deficit in memory is due to a failure of retrieval on the basis of a theoretical distinction among processes of encoding, storage, and retrieval. While this may represent a potentially more specific description of the memory problem associated with increased age, it does not qualify as a true explanation without additional information. We would have to know why retrieval processes are affected and other processes are not (e.g., because the retrieval cues are lost due to atrophy of neurons, because the "catalog" for information storage has a finite capacity, etc.), and ideally some statement should be provided as to how the retrieval processes became defective as the individual grew older.

Despite the difficulties associated with theorizing in adult development, it still must be concluded that the attempt is worth the effort. The literature in this area is currently so diverse and chaotic that it is sometimes difficult to discern any progress, or even any real sense of continuity. Theories that would integrate and organize even a small portion of this literature, and perhaps serve to suggest avenues of useful investigation, could only improve this situation. One must expect the early attempts at theorizing to be rather primitive, and for the theories to evolve quite rapidly when they are first introduced. As with other disciplines, however, the abandonment and revision of theories will probably proceed at a much slower rate once the field is more developed.

Replacing the Age Variable

One of the major goals of theories in aging is to identify variables that can be used to replace the variable of chronological age. While the age variable is a very powerful index for classifying behavior (perhaps even the most power-ful individual-difference variable), it does not by itself lead to explanation. The discovery that a particular variable is significantly related to age may be interesting as a descriptive fact, but it provides no information about why that relationship exists. As a number of authors have pointed out (e.g., Baltes & Goulet, 1971; Baltes, Reese, & Nesselroade, 1978; Birren, 1959; Botwinick, 1978; Kuhlen, 1963; Wohlwill, 1970), age is not a causal variable; the passage of time in and of itself is responsible for nothing. Explanations of changes associated with age or the passage of time must therefore rely on variables that exert their effects over time, not time itself. In this regard, Wohlwill (1970) has suggested that chronological age is best conceptualized as a part of the dependent variable, a dimension along which change is measured, rather than as an independent variable.

The great majority of past research in the psychology of aging has been descriptive, as is fitting for the early stages of a developing science. Wohlwill (1970) was absolutely correct in asserting that it is a "... truism that it is essential to have an adequate knowledge of a phenomenon before one can set about explaining it" (p. 54). Eventually, however, scientists do hope to discover the causes of the phenomena they observe. In order to do this in developmental psychology, the chronological age variable must be replaced with an experimental variable. That variable can then be manipulated under controlled conditions to determine whether the differences produced by the variable are similar to the differences associated with increased age. After the examination of many such variables the causal variables can ultimately be selected to be incorporated in the interpretation of the differences associated with age. It is this type of reasoning that led Birren and Renner (1977) to make what seems to be a paradoxical statement for a developmental psychologist: "In a rigorously experimental sense, age must be approached in research as a variable that ultimately must be eliminated" (p. 26).

Dimensions for Theory Classification

Throughout much of the remainder of this book evidence will be examined in an attempt to rule out certain types of explanation for observed age differences in behavior. As a means of bringing some order into this theory-evaluation process, the present section outlines some of the more important dimensions which can be used for classifying theories of aging.

Rather broad terms will be used to describe the theoretical dimensions because of a belief that the type of data currently available in behavioral research is not precise enough to warrant very fine distinctions among theoretical alternatives. The notion that even results from studies in experimental psychology, with their legendary rigor and extreme control, have limited resolution for distinguishing among possible theories might be considered heresy in some circles (but see Broadbent, 1971, for a viewpoint similar to that expressed here). However, even a cursory survey reveals that very few topic areas in psychology are well enough understood to allow precise, quantitative predictions in the place of broad, qualitative statements. Theories will naturally continue to be elaborated to the limits of the theorist's ingenuity. What must be resisted is the temptation to assume that because a few general and testable implications have been supported, all of the finer detailed predictions, which often cannot be precisely tested, are also supported. Adherence to this caution will limit the specificity of the conclusions and probably make exact predictions impossible, but the generalizations that are made can usually be stated with considerable confidence.

The first classification dimension to be considered is whether the observed group differences are primarily due to maturational or environmental processes. Maturational processes are those determined by the biological characteristics of the species and which occur solely as a function of the length of time the organism is in a normal environment. These types of processes, although subject to slight variation in qualitative pattern and time of onset due to within-species genetic differences, should be approximately the same in all members of a given species across a wide range of environmental conditions.

In contrast, environmental processes are those factors often associated with advancing age but which are ultimately attributable to sources outside the organism. As used here, this alternative may include such broad factors as climate, culture, and nutrition, as well as such specific factors as living through the winter of 1978, watching televised coverage of astronauts walking on the surface of the moon, or eating a McDonald's hamburger. We learned in the last chapter that separation of the influence of maturational and environmental factors is extremely difficult. Moreover, in many cases the two factors may interact with one another such that the resulting behavior is a joint function of specific maturational processes and environmental conditions. In principle, however, the fundamental issue is whether specific experience is important; nearly any type of experience should suffice according to the maturational perspective, whereas a specific type of experience is assumed to be necessary with the environmental perspective.

A second dimension that will be used for classifying theories of aging is related to the distinction between competence and performance. Competence refers to the individual's capability or potential, while performance designates the actual behavior that the individual produces. Cohen (1977), using the terms "can" and "do" instead of competence and performance, has commented on the confusion surrounding these concepts:

> It may seem unnecessary to stress the obvious fact that while "do" implies "can do," and "can't" implies "don't," the reverse does not hold. "Can do" does not imply "do," and "don't" does not imply "can't." In many areas of research psychologists fail to make clear whether they are investigating norms or limits, habits or capacities. (p. 93)

Observation of an individual's normal performance may therefore be informative only about the individual's minimum capacities; it might tell us nothing about the maximum of which he or she is capable.

The manner in which the competence-performance distinction is related to a classification dimension for categorizing aging theories concerns the degree to which a theory assumes that performance mirrors competence. If the theory makes a rigid distinction between performance and competence, for example by assuming that age differences are attributable to a differential use of particular strategies with no underlying difference in actual potential, then the theory would be placed on one end of this continuum. However, if the theory makes no provision for a distinction between performance and competence, and implicitly assumes that typical performance is equivalent to maximal performance for all age groups, then the theory would be placed on the other end of the continuum.

The third major classification dimension is essentially a general versus specific dimension. If a theory of aging utilizes a general mechanism that can account for a wide variety of aging phenomena, it would be placed near the general end of this dimension. On the other hand, if the theory is concerned with a very specific mechanism that applies to only a few structures or functions and affects only a limited subset of possible measures, it would be placed near the specific end of the dimension.

There are obviously other dimensions that might be proposed to help classify aging theories, but the three listed above appear to represent some of the most fundamental, and potentially resolvable, theoretical issues at the present time. Because of its current popularity among many developmental psychologists, the distinction between qualitative and quantitative differences deserves special comment. Some researchers have attempted to determine whether adults of varying ages perform tasks in a different fashion (i.e., exhibit a qualitative difference), or in the same manner but at different levels of proficiency (i.e., exhibit a quantitative difference). Although sometimes meaningful, this distinction is often misleading because a qualitative shift would likely produce quantitative differences in the effectiveness of various performance components, and it is also probable that a quantitative change at an elementary level would lead to qualitative differences in the processes employed at higher levels. The qualitative-quantitative debate might therefore be considered analogous to the controversy about whether the chicken or the egg came first, and it does not seem fruitful to engage in this type of speculation at the current time.

In the following sections two broad theories are discussed to illustrate the three dimensions outlined above in a concrete fashion. The theories are patterned on actual speculations from researchers in the field of adult development, but it is unlikely that any individual researcher would subscribe fully to either of the theories as presented. They have been extensively modified and elaborated in such a manner that the current versions probably do not represent the views of any of the original theorists.

At the outset several limitations of the following discussion should be pointed out. One is that these theories, perhaps even more than is the case with most theories, are necessarily incomplete, vague, and undoubtedly wrong in many respects. Nevertheless, they should prove useful for illustrating some of the approaches that one might take in theorizing about aging phenomena, and naturally many variations of these theories could be proposed and one of these variations might ultimately prove more successful than the original theory. The second limitation to be recognized in the following discussion is that although the theories are portrayed as though they were mutually exclusive, it is almost certainly the case that many abilities involve a combination of determinants and thus both theoretical perspectives may be partially true. As Baltes and Willis (1977, p. 143) have noted, it is unrealistic to expect a "monolithic, single explanation" of many aging phenomena; an assessment of the relative contribution of different determinants would often be much more realistic than attempting to identify a single, absolute cause. And finally, just as one should not expect a given phenomenon to have but a single cause, one should not expect many different phenomena to be determined by the same combination of causal factors. Aging phenomena must be considered to be multidimensional in manifestation as well in causality.

Two Illustrative Theories

Neural-Noise Theory

One theory of aging processes might be termed the neural-noise theory in that it assumes that most decrements associated with increased age are ultimately attributable to an age-related reduction in effective signal-to-noise ratio within the nervous system. There are a variety of possible causes for this postulated increase in neural noise, e.g., loss of neurons, decreased cerebral blood flow, increased randomness in neural activity, etc., but all lead to the assumption that signals are less discriminable in the nervous system of older adults relative to younger adults. The consequence of this reduced signal-to-noise ratio is that older adults will have higher sensory thresholds than younger adults (because of the need for more intense stimulation to counteract the increased internal noise level) and will be slower in nearly all processes than younger adults (because of the need to integrate stimulation over a longer period of time to attain equivalent clarity).

In addition to these two direct implications of the neural-noise theory, there are also a number of indirect, or secondary, implications. For example, if sensory thresholds are higher in the older adult, it is possible that some sensory stimulation never enters the nervous system and thus the older individual might be handicapped by receiving less environmental information than the younger individual. In certain situations the differential availability of information across age groups may hinder performance in complex activities where that information is required.

Quantitative and qualitative deficits in higher cognitive processes might also be produced by a generalized speed loss. As an illustration, if the solution to a problem requires the simultaneous awareness of many prior steps, the elderly individual may be handicapped because his or her slower rate of working results in the earlier steps being unavailable by the time the later step is reached. In this case both the quality as well as the quantity of the output will be reduced with increased age. Generalized speed losses may also lead to poorer memory performance (because less time is available for organization, elaboration, or rehearsal of information), and to inefficiencies when attention must be divided among several different sources of information (because the time available for each source and for switching between sources is less than that of younger adults).

Although this description is necessarily vague because it contains no reference to any specific research area, the major characteristics of the neural-noise theory are apparent. For example, it would be classified along the maturational end of the maturation-environment continuum because the increase in neural noise is presumed to be a biological consequence of normal aging, and the specific type of environmental experience is unimportant as long as it does not affect the rate of neural deterioration. Further, the neural-noise theory would be classified on the competence end of the performance-competence dimension as the primary cause of most aging deficits is assumed to be the competence-limiting factor of increased neural noise, and not some factor that merely affects performance. And finally, the neural-noise theory is assumed to be quite general, applying to a variety of sensory, motor, and cognitive deficits, and thus it would be classified towards the general end of the general-specific continuum.

Disuse Theory

One of a class of theories that emphasize social or psychological rather than biological causes of aging differences is the disuse theory. This type of theory recognizes the great differences in interests, attitudes, and experiences that exist across various age groups, and assumes that these differences can be at least partially responsible for the decrements observed in many aspects of behavior. The mechanism by which these various factors exert their influence on behavior is by channeling the individual's interests and experiences in certain directions to the exclusion of other directions. That is, as an adult grows older there may not be a loss of any initial ability, but the pattern of daily activity and the nature of one's interests almost certainly changes. The disuse theory assumes that this differential experience and responsiveness to reinforcements is responsible for many of the reported age differences in behavior.

One of the fundamental assumptions behind this approach seems to be that practice or experience is necessary for an ability to develop or be maintained; without such use, a function will atrophy in the same manner as a muscle which has been incapacitated. The specific form of the atrophy can be expected to vary across abilities; in some it might be evident in the use of inefficient strategies, whereas in others it might be reflected by an inappropriate focus of attention or a variety of other specific mechanisms.

Another assumption of the disuse theory is that a young adult, perhaps because of recent exposure to the educational system, is equally practiced or experienced in nearly all abilities, and that as he or she begins to develop special skills for particular vocations certain of these abilities are used more frequently than others. Over a period of many years this differential frequency of usage is thought to be responsible for the decline in unused abilities reflected in age-related performance decrements observed in psychometric tests and psychological experiments.

In terms of the classification dimensions discussed earlier, the disuse theory would clearly be placed on the environmental end of the maturation-environment dimension. The presumed causes of the age group differences are differential environmental experiences, not intrinsic maturational factors. Categorization along the performance-competence dimension depends upon whether one views the atrophy as irreversible or potentially remedial. If exposure to a new set of environmental experiences can lead to the elimination of the age differences, then the theory would be placed at the performance end of the continuum. However, if no amount of new experience can succeed in eliminating the age differences, then the differences would have to be considered competency-based, and not simply a limitation of performance. The version of the disuse theory to be considered here will assume that the absence of practice has not led to any structural change within the nervous system, and thus it would be classified at the performance end of the continuum.

The disuse theory is also somewhat difficult to place along the general-specific dimension because while the theory may apply to all aspects of behavior, it can only account for deficits in abilities that are unpracticed in older adults. In other words, the theory is general, but has plausibility only for those abilities that are not used in daily living.

Forewarning

We can anticipate some of the discussions of later chapters by stating that at the present time there is little concrete evidence to distinguish between the neural-noise and disuse theories. Either the appropriate research has not been conducted, or the results available thus far have been inconsistent and even contradictory. This is actually a sad commentary on the state of theoretical development in adult cognition since the neural-noise and disuse theories were specifically selected as examples because of their distinct positions on three important dimensions.

Despite the lack of definitive evidence at the present time, it is still useful to examine research in the context of theoretical perspectives if for no other reason than to identify the weaknesses of the current evidence for the purposes of making theoretical distinctions. While no firm conclusions will be drawn, the final chapter will summarize the major evidence relevant to the two illustrative theories, and also speculate about what is needed in order to increase the rate of theoretical development in adult cognition.

Aging Defined by Theory

It may be surprising to some readers that no definition of aging, the fundamental topic of this book, has yet been offered. The reason for this delay has been to emphasize the role of one's theoretical assumptions in determining the definition of aging. Many of the common definitions of aging contain such phrases as "progressive deterioration," "decrease in reactivity," or "reduced power of adaptation" that clearly imply a particular type of perspective that Schaie (1977) has termed the irreversible-decrement model. Alternative perspectives such as what Schaie (1977) calls the stability model, or the decrement-with-compensation model, would have led to quite different definitions, and thus it is rather difficult to provide a theoretically neutral definition of aging. Birren and Renner (1977) perhaps come the closest in such a definition, as they specifically selected one that "does not imply an exclusively biological, environmental, or social causality, and keeps the door open for the study of the incremental as well as the decremental changes in functions which occur over the life span" (p. 4). Their definition is as follows:

> ... aging refers to the regular changes that occur in mature genetically representative organisms living under representative environmental conditions as they advance in chronological age. (Birren & Renner, 1977, p. 4)

The Birren and Renner definition is particularly suitable in the present context because it can be used with both the neural-noise and the disuse theories. Although the two theories considered separately would lead to quite different interpretations of the aging process, the definition provided by Birren and Renner has the advantage of describing aging in a manner acceptable to nearly all theoretical perspectives.

Summary

Theories serve to provide structure and direction for research. Since the current literature in adult cognition is nearly devoid of both of these attributes, it is argued that theories are essential for progress in this area. Theories can be developed within the context of adult development, or imported from related disciplines with constant-age individuals. In either case the theory must account for the processes of change occurring across the life span and not just the processes themselves.

Three dimensions were identified for classifying developmental theories: environmental versus maturational, performance versus competence, and general versus specific. Two theories representing positions at different ends of the three continua were described to illustrate some of the potential differences among classes of theories. Finally, the problems associated with providing a theoretically neutral definition of aging were discussed, and a definition provided by Birren and Renner (1977) was selected as the best available description of the processes of aging.

4. Psychometric Intelligence

Intelligence tests have the unique distinction of simultaneously being one of the most successful, and the most controversial, of psychology's accomplishments. The controversy and the interest have carried over into research on adult development as nearly half of the psychological studies published in the *Journal of Gerontology* in recent years have been concerned with intellectual and cognitive functioning (Abrahams, Hoyer, Elias, & Bradigan, 1975). This is not surprising considering the high value placed on intellectual competence in modern society, and the fact that much of the available research has been interpreted to suggest that intelligence declines more or less continuously beginning at early maturity.

The term "mental test" was first used by Cattell (1890) to refer to a battery of sensory and motor measures designed to assess mental power. Perhaps because of the nature of the subtests, e.g., two-point tactile threshold, reaction time, strength of hand grip, etc., Cattell's battery was not very successful at predicting performance on intellectual activities such as school work. It was Binet (e.g., Binet & Henri, 1895; Binet & Simon, 1905) who introduced more cognitive subtests into intelligence test batteries, many of which are still used in modern intelligence tests.

The first large-scale application of intelligence tests to an adult population occurred in World War I, when psychologists were asked to help classify young men for various military activities. The primary classification test, the Army Alpha, consisted of eight timed tests assessing a variety of abilities ranging from general information and vocabulary to series completion and analogical reasoning. One of the most surprising findings from this enormous project was that the composite intelligence measure declined systematically with increasing age beginning at about age 25. Some typical data are illustrated in Figure 4.1. (The ordinate in this and most other figures throughout the book is the percentage that the mean of each age group is of the maximum performance across all age groups. The advantage of this form of presentation is that studies employing different dependent variables can be compared in an intuitively meaningful manner.)

Although the functions of Figure 4.1 seem fairly definitive, particularly in light of the large number of individuals involved, the researchers interpreting these results were reluctant to conclude that there was a true negative relationship between age and intelligence. For example, Yerkes (1921) suggested that a selection bias may have been operating such that, for a variety of reasons, the older individuals in the military sample came from a less intelligent segment of the population than the younger individuals.

Differential selection was not a problem in a later large-scale study utilizing the same Army Alpha test. Jones and Conrad (1933) administered the test to a cross-section of individuals from rural New England communities, in many

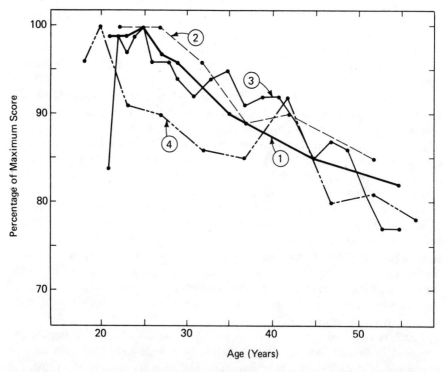

Figure 4.1. Scores on the Army Alpha Intelligence Test at various ages expressed as a percentage of the maximum score across all ages. Numbers refer to different samples: 1 = 15,385 soldiers (adapted from Table 366, Yerkes, 1921); 2 = 1,192 soldiers (adapted from Table 368, Yerkes, 1921); 3 = 5,742 soldiers (adapted from Table 369, Yerkes, 1921); and 4 = community residents (Jones & Conrad, 1933).

cases testing nearly the entire adult population of a community. The major results from this study, plotted along with the World War I results in Figure 4.1, were very consistent with those from the military testings. Jones and Conrad were quite thorough in considering the plausibility of alternative explanations for their results, e.g., differential selection, motivation, sensory acuity, etc., and in the end felt compelled to conclude that intelligence did indeed decline with increased age.

This same trend of a negative relationship between age and intelligence score was reported in many subsequent studies employing a variety of intelligence tests (e.g., Foster & Taylor, 1920; Miles & Miles, 1932; Mursell, 1929; Raven, 1948; Vincent, 1952; Wechsler, 1939). Despite the very similar findings in many independent studies, the relationship between adult age and intelligence has been a topic of great controversy since the very first Army Alpha results. For example, criticism has been directed at the speeded and child-oriented nature of most intelligence tests, and at the failure to account for age-related changes in educational background, interests, and motivation when interpreting the results of such studies. In recent years much of the debate has focused upon the apparent discrepancy between results obtained with cross-sectional methods and longitudinal methods. (For an illustration of the current version of this controversy see the exchange between Baltes and Schaie on the one hand (e.g., Baltes & Schaie, 1974, 1976; Schaie, 1974; Schaie & Parham, 1977) and Horn & Donaldson (1976, 1977) on the other hand.)

The viewpoint adopted here is that many of the issues of concern to earlier researchers were confusing primarily because a variety of different definitions of intelligence were employed. It is believed that much of the confusion and controversy surrounding these issues is eliminated when distinctions are made concerning the particular type of intelligence being investigated. As a means of making this distinction, the next section briefly examines some of the ways in which intelligence has been defined by psychologists in the past.

Definition of Intelligence

It has been said that intelligence is one of those concepts that everyone understands and yet no one can adequately define. This is not to say that no definitions have been proposed, but rather that no definition has been found that has proved satisfactory to all parties. Examples of such limited definitions are: "ability to learn," "ability to organize experience and recognize relationships," "effective utilization of stored information," "capability of modifying the environment," and even "capacity to appreciate Shakespeare's plays." Still more difficult than the problem of defining intelligence is the problem of measuring it. As should be apparent from the above sample of definitions, obtaining behavioral indices of such a global concept like intelligence is no easy task.

Either because of a desire to measure many different expressions of intelligence, or merely because a heterogeneous sample of behaviors produces greater validity, most intelligence tests have traditionally been comprised of a number of subtests, each calling for a slightly different type of activity. The overall intelligence score is then either a weighted or unweighted aggregate of the various subtest scores.

Within the field of intelligence testing there is some dispute about whether the various subtests are merely different measures of the same kind of intelligence, or measures of different kinds of intelligence. This debate is of only peripheral interest here, but two observations pertinent to this issue are relevant to the present discussion. The first is that at any given age the various subtests are generally highly correlated with one another. This is rather surprising in view of the diverse nature of many of the subtests, and it has been taken as evidence for the existence of a common factor of general intelligence. The second observation, that the various subtests exhibit quite different developmental trends, seems to suggest that intelligence is not unitary and that there are different, functionally independent, forms of intelligence.

Taken together, these observations indicate that while the composite intelligence score has some justification for being considered a measure of global intelligence, its meaning may be substantially different at various portions of the life span because the same composite score can be produced by many different combinations of subtest scores. If some of the subtest abilities are declining with age while others are improving, the composite measure might be very misleading in indicating no age differences in overall intelligence. To the extent that the various subtests differ in their developmental trends, therefore, it seems unreasonable to attempt to make interpretations about the relationship between age and intelligence on the basis of a single composite measure of intelligence.

In fact, the discovery that the component abilities of an intelligence test do exhibit differential age trends was one of the earliest, and is still one of the best supported, findings in the field of adult developmental psychology (e.g., Beeson, 1920; Foster & Taylor, 1920; Jones & Conrad, 1933; Miles, 1933; Sorenson, 1938; Weisenburg, Roe, & McBride, 1936; Willoughby, 1927). The following sections discuss some of the more recent evidence concerning this differential decline.

Before leaving the topic of the definition of intelligence, the application of factor analysis techniques to the problem of identifying the organization of intelligence should be briefly mentioned. The purpose of factor analysis is to examine the relationships among a large number of measures in an attempt to identify a smaller number of related factors, components, or clusters. This technique would thus seem to be ideal for examining the structure of intelligence at various developmental periods by simply comparing the factors identified at each age level. Unfortunately, factor analysis has not proven very successful in studies of adult intellectual development as there has been very little consistency in the results from different investigations. Some investigators have reported that there is little change in factorial structure across the adult life span (e.g., Cohen, 1957; Riegel & Riegel, 1962; Weiner, 1964; Wilson, DeFries, McClearn, Vandenberg, Johnson, & Rashad, 1975), others have reported changes but some have claimed that the change is towards fewer factors (or higher weightings on dominant factors) with increased age (e.g., Balinsky, 1941; Baltes, Cornelius, Spiro, Nesselroade, & Willis, 1980; Berger, Bernstein, Klein, Cohen & Lucas, 1964; Cunningham & Birren, 1980; Green & Berkowitz, 1964; Leinert & Crott, 1964; McHugh & Owens, 1954), and some have claimed that the change is towards more factors (e.g., Radcliffe, 1966). Factor analysis techniques offer a promising perspective on the issue of changing intellectual structure, but a combination of inconsistent methods and inadequate data have resulted in limited contributions thus far.

Analyses of Component Abilities

Because the Wechsler Adult Intelligence Scale (WAIS) is the most frequently used intelligence test with adults, it has the greatest amount of data relevant to the issue of differential decline of component abilities. For this reason we will use the WAIS as our prototypical intelligence test, and will examine the developmental trends in each of its 11 subtests separately. Such a subtest analysis is actually essential in order to understand how intelligence is measured in the WAIS, as Wechsler's (1958) definition of intelligence, like those mentioned earlier, offers no clear indication of how the measurement of intelligence is accomplished, i.e., "Intelligence operationally defined is the aggregate or global capacity of the individual to act purposefully, to think rationally, and to deal effectively with his environment" (1958, p. 7).

Following the discussion of the WAIS subtests, two additional subtests often included in other global tests of intelligence, i.e., series completion and analogical tests of reasoning, will also be examined in terms of their developmental trends in adulthood.

The results of several studies with at least 100 individuals across a wide range of ages will be displayed for each subtest. Because we will be attempting to draw rather broad conclusions, the general pattern across all studies will be emphasized rather than the results of any particular study. Fortunately, the data are reasonably consistent and it is not difficult to discern major trends. Since many of the same individuals contributed data in all subtests, it will also be possible to make some tentative statements about the relative magnitudes of age differences for the various subtests. These should be interpreted with great caution, however, because it is possible that alternative tests of the same ability might yield quite different age trends.

Verbal Abilities

Four of the WAIS subtests, Vocabulary, Information, Comprehension, and Similarities, can be described as measuring some type of verbal ability. Since the age trends in these subtests are also fairly similar, they are grouped together in the present section to facilitate discussion.

The Vocabulary subtest in the WAIS involves the examinee being asked to provide the meaning of 40 words. The responses are scored on a 3-point scale based on the quality of the definitions.

Performance on the WAIS Vocabulary test as a function of adult age is illustrated in Figure 4.2. Although there is considerable variation in these data, it is apparent that the scores do not decline systematically with increased age. Other tests of vocabulary yield very similar results as many investigators have reported that vocabulary either remains stable or increases across the life span (e.g., Foulds & Raven, 1948; Gardner & Monge, 1977; Horn & Cattell, 1966; Jones & Conrad, 1933; W. Miles, 1933; Schaie, 1958; Thorndike & Gallup, 1944; Weisenburg et al., 1936).

The WAIS Information subtest consists of 29 questions of general information. Different questions relate to facts about one's culture, to geographical relationships among countries, and to the author, theme, and identity of various written works.

Age functions for the WAIS Information subtest are displayed in Figure 4.3, where it can be seen that there is little or no trend associated with increased age. A similar stability across the age span was reported in the

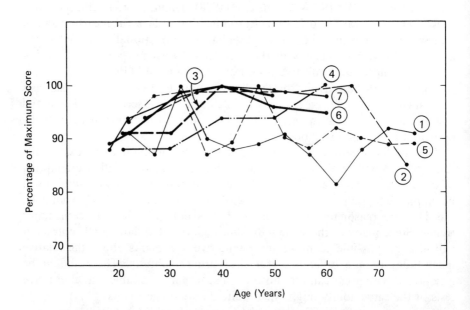

Figure 4.2. WAIS Vocabulary score at various ages expressed as a percentage of the maximum score across all ages. Numbers refer to different samples: 1 = adapted from Berkowitz (1953); 2 = adapted from Botwinick & Storandt (1974a); 3 = adapted from Goldfarb (1941)—females; 4 = adapted from Goldfarb (1941)—males; 5 = adapted from Howell (1955); 6 = adapted from Wechsler (1958)—females; and 7 = adapted from Wechsler (1958)—males.

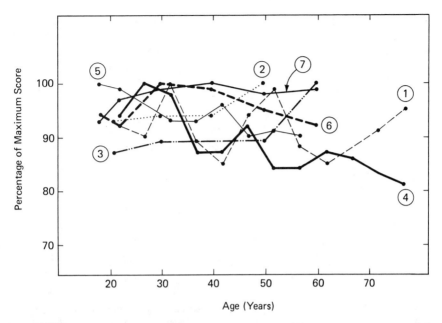

Figure 4.3. WAIS Information score at various ages expressed as a percentage of the maximum score across all ages. Numbers refer to different samples: 1 = adapted from Berkowitz (1953); 2 = adapted from Goldfarb (1941)—females; 3 = adapted from Goldfarb (1941)—males; 4 = adapted from Howell (1955); 5 = adapted from Wechsler (1944); 6 = adapted from Wechsler (1958)—females; and 7 = adapted from Wechsler (1958)—males.

General Information subtest of the Army Alpha by Jones and Conrad (1933). Gardner and Monge (1977) have also reported age invariance in tests of information about transportation, death and disease, and finance.

The WAIS Comprehension subtest consists of 14 questions relating to common sense information, or interpretation of familiar proverbs. The data in Figure 4.4 indicate that performance on this test exhibits little difference until the age of 50 or 60, but may decrease beyond that age. Foster and Taylor (1920) also reported little or no cross-sectional age decline in a similar test, although Jones and Conrad (1933) found a substantial decline in the timed comprehension test from the Army Alpha.

The Similarities subtest is a type of verbal analogies test in that the examinee is given two words and is asked to state a way in which the two are similar. Thirteen word pairs are presented, with the scoring based on the quality of the responses. The age functions for this test, presented in Figure 4.5, seem to suggest a slight reduction with increased age. A much steeper cross-sectional age decline has been reported in verbal analogies tests involving greater amounts of reasoning and abstraction (e.g., Garfield & Blek, 1952; Gilbert, 1935; Horn & Cattell, 1966; Jones & Conrad, 1933; Mason & Ganzler, 1964; Owens, 1953; Riegel, 1959; Weisenburg et al., 1936; Willoughby, 1927).

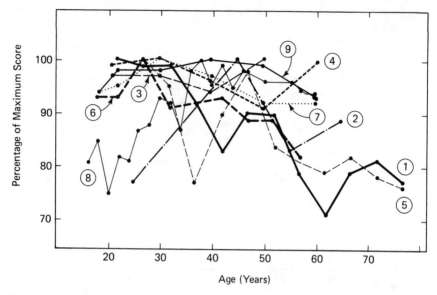

Figure 4.4. WAIS Comprehension score at various ages expressed as a percentage of the maximum score across all ages. Numbers refer to different samples: 1 = adapted from Berkowitz (1953); 2 = adapted from Botwinick & Storandt (1974a); 3 = adapted from Goldfarb (1941)—females; 4 = adapted from Goldfarb (1941)—males; 5 = adapted from Howell (1955); 6 = adapted from Wechsler (1944); 7 = adapted from Wechsler (1958)—females; 8 = adapted from Wechsler (1958)—males; and 9 = adapted from Whiteman & Jastak (1957).

In some respects the stability of vocabulary performance (and other measures of verbal ability) across the life span is rather surprising. Conrad (1930), Jones (1959), and Wechsler (1958) have all noted that if one assumes that learning ability remains unimpaired throughout the life span, an individual aged 65 should score much higher than an individual aged 25 on tests of stored information merely because the older individual has had 40 more years of acquisition opportunity. The absence of such an improvement may be a reflection of a decrease in the quality of environmental stimulation, or a reduction in learning ability, in later life. In either case, it appears as though most existing tests of verbal ability reflect the cumulative effects of stored experience more than current status, and thus they may be more indicative of past attainments rather than present ability (cf. Bromley, 1974; Jones, 1959).

This interpretation suggests that other, more demanding, tests of verbal ability might reveal substantially different aging trends. In fact, several studies have found sizable age decrements with alternative measures of verbal ability. For instance, older individuals report less words of a particular type, e.g., those beginning with the letter *S*, in timed tests of verbal fluency than younger individuals (e.g., Bilash & Zubek, 1960; Birren, 1955; Birren, Riegel, & Morrison, 1962; Foster & Taylor, 1920; Riegel, 1959; Schaie, 1958; Schaie, Rosenthal, & Perlman, 1953; Schaie & Strother, 1968a; Strother, Schaie, & Horst, 1957).

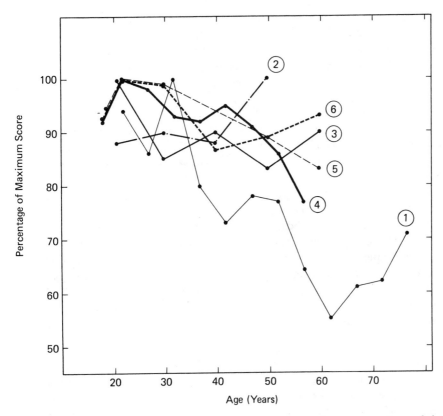

Figure 4.5. WAIS Similarities score at various ages expressed as a percentage of the maximum score across all ages. Numbers refer to different samples: 1 = adapted from Berkowitz (1953); 2 = adapted from Goldfarb (1941)—females; 3 = adapted from Goldfarb (1941)—males; 4 = adapted from Wechsler (1944); 5 = adapted from Wechsler (1958)—females; and 6 = adapted from Wechsler (1958)—males.

It has also been suggested that while older adults are able to provide an adequate definition of many words, the quality of their definitions may be lower than that of younger adults. Unfortunately, the evidence with respect to this latter issue is rather mixed, as some studies have reported such an age difference in the quality of definitions (e.g., Botwinick & Storandt, 1974b; Looft, 1970), but others failed to find statistically significant differences (e.g., Storck & Looft, 1973) or failed to find a significant age by scoring method (quality) interaction (e.g., Botwinick, West, & Storandt, 1975).

Finally, it appears that when people are asked to do something more than merely define the words, such as classify them (e.g., Riegel, 1959) or perform verbal analogies (e.g., Farmer, McLean, Sparks, & O'Connell, 1978; Gilbert, 1935; Horn & Cattell, 1966; Jones & Conrad, 1933; Owens, 1953; Riegel, 1959; Willoughby, 1927), pronounced age differences are again apparent.

This mixed assortment of results concerning the relationship between age and verbal abilities suggests that the existing tests of vocabulary, information, etc., may not be very satisfactory measures of actual verbal ability. Perhaps an assessment of active, as opposed to passive, ability would lead to better evaluation. There are at least two methods by which such an active vocabulary assessment might be obtained, and one of these has already been applied in an adult development context. The technique already tried involves analyzing the written works (e.g., letters, diaries, journals, etc.) of individuals at several different periods in their life. Smith (1957a, 1957b) and Dennis (1960) have explored this technique, but no definitive conclusions about adult changes in active vocabulary are yet possible because the number of individuals studied with the technique thus far has been quite small (i.e., from 2 to 14).

An alternative technique suggested by Howes (1971) consists of examining oral rather than written verbal behavior. Howes proposed tape-recording samples of an individual's speech in a particular situation and then analyzing the range and frequency of words in the speech sample to estimate the size of the individual's active vocabulary. This technique could also be used to determine the degree of redundancy in the speech sample by comparing the relative frequency of specific word sequences with the normative frequency of those sequences in the speech of a large population. More research is needed in this area as it would be desirable to determine whether alternative methods of assessing verbal ability will yield the same pattern of results as that reported with existing measures.

Numerical Abilities

The Arithmetic subtest of the WAIS consists of 14 simple arithmetic word problems, with bonuses allowed for rapid responses in some of the problems. Figure 4.6 indicates that arithmetic ability is fairly stable through about age 50, after which time a performance reduction may be beginning. Other tests of arithmetic have yielded a mixture of results, with some indicating little difference with age (e.g., Bilash & Zubek, 1960; Brown & Ghiselli, 1949; Glanzer et al. 1958; Kamin, 1957; Schaie et al. 1953; Schaie & Strother, 1968a, 1968b; Sorenson, 1933), and others moderate difference in favor of young adults (e.g., Beeson, 1920; Birren & Botwinick, 1951; Gardner & Monge, 1977; Jones & Conrad, 1933). Bromley (1974, p. 188) has suggested that tests emphasizing mechanical computation tend to produce stable age functions, whereas those requiring thoughtful reasoning tend to produce age-related declines. This interpretation does not seem to fit the WAIS data very well, as the WAIS Arithmetic test seems to require a moderate amount of thoughtful reasoning and yet it does not produce a very dramatic cross-sectional age decline. Nevertheless, the mechanical-thoughtful distinction may be useful in characterizing much of the remaining data on age relationships in numerical abilities.

Memory Abilities

The WAIS Digit Span test involves testing individuals with the longest series of digits they can repeat without error in both the original sequence, and in a reversed sequence. The total score is the sum of the maximum

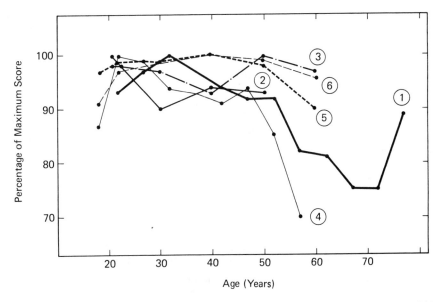

Figure 4.6. WAIS Arithmetic score at various ages expressed as a percentage of the maximum score across all ages. Numbers refer to different samples: 1 = adapted from Berkowitz (1953); 2 = adapted from Goldfarb (1941)—females; 3 = adapted from Goldfarb (1941)—males; 4 = adapted from Wechsler (1944); 5 = adapted from Wechsler (1958)—females; and 6 = adapted from Wechsler (1958)—males.

sequence correctly reported in the forward and backward orders. Figure 4.7 indicates that performance on this test is negatively associated with increased age, such that an individual in his or her 50s is, on the average, performing at about 80% of the level of an individual in his or her 20s. Similar results with other memory span tests have been reported by Botwinick and Storandt (1974a), Dirken (1972), Gilbert (1935), Heron and Chown (1967), Muhs, Hooper and Papalia-Finley (1979), and Trembly and O'Connor (1966).

Spatial Abilities

Four of the WAIS subtests, i.e., Object Assembly, Picture Completion, Picture Arrangement, and Block Design, can be described as involving spatial abilities.

The Object Assembly subtest involves the examinee attempting to arrange the parts of a figure to make a complete pattern in a manner similar to a jigsaw puzzle. Four patterns are presented with time limits of either 120 or 180 seconds each, and bonuses allowed for rapid responses. The age functions are illustrated in Figure 4.8. Notice that there is a fairly constant performance difference of about 5% per decade beginning at about age 25 or 30.

The Picture Completion subtest of the WAIS requires identification of the element missing from a particular picture. Examinees are allowed 20 seconds for each of 21 pictures. Figure 4.9 indicates that the cross-sectional age

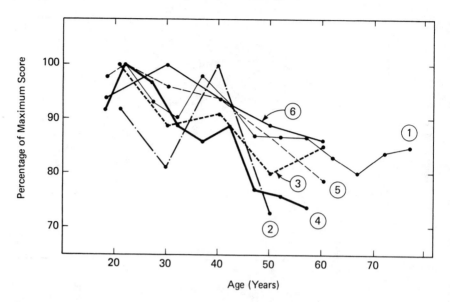

Figure 4.7. WAIS Digit Span score at various ages expressed as a percentage of the maximum score across all ages. Numbers refer to different samples: 1 = adapted from Berkowitz (1953); 2 = adapted from Goldfarb (1941)—females; 3 = adapted from Goldfarb (1941)—males; 4 = adapted from Wechsler (1944); 5 = adapted from Wechsler (1958)—females; and 6 = adapted from Wechsler (1958)—males.

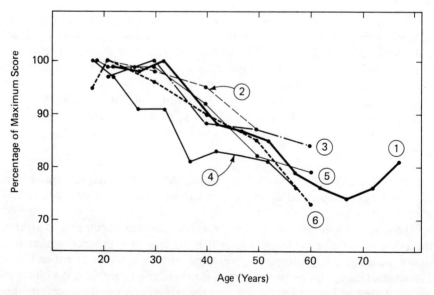

Figure 4.8. WAIS Object Assembly score at various ages expressed as a percentage of the maximum score across all ages. Numbers refer to different samples: 1 = adapted from Berkowitz (1953); 2 = adapted from Goldfarb (1941)—females; 3 = adapted from Goldfarb (1941)—males; 4 = adapted from Wechsler (1944); 5 = adapted from Wechsler (1958)—females; and 6 = adapted from Wechsler (1958)—males.

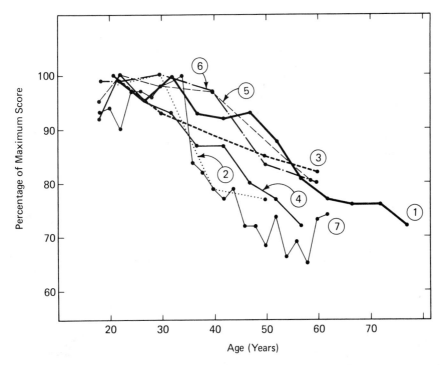

Figure 4.9. WAIS Picture Completion score at various ages expressed as a percentage of the maximum score across all ages. Numbers refer to different samples: 1 = adapted from Berkowitz (1953); 2 = adapted from Goldfarb (1941)—females; 3 = adapted from Goldfarb (1941)—males; 4 = adapted from Wechsler (1944); 5 = adapted from Wechsler (1958)—females; 6 = adapted from Wechsler (1958)—males; and 7 = adapted from Whiteman & Jastak (1957).

declines on this test are very similar to those in the Object Assembly test as the rate of cross-sectional decline is again about 5% per decade.

The WAIS Block Design subtest involves the examinee attempting to arrange a number of patterned blocks to match a specific design. Ten design problems are presented, with a bonus allowed for quick responses on the most difficult problems. The age functions for this test are illustrated in Figure 4.10. The rate of decline is approximately 8% per decade.

The WAIS Picture Arrangement subtest requires the examinee to arrange a series of pictures into a sequence that conveys a meaningful story. Eight series are presented, with a time limit and a quick-response bonus for each series. Figure 4.11 exhibits the age functions from this subtest. Notice that the cross-sectional age declines are quite steep, averaging over 10% per decade, or about 1% per year.

The finding that older adults are generally poorer than young adults on tests of visual or spatial abilities has been repeatedly confirmed with a variety of other psychometric tests (e.g., Arenberg, 1978; 1982; Berg, Hertzog, & Hunt, 1982; Bilash & Zubek, 1960; Bromley, 1966; Chown, 1961; Fozard &

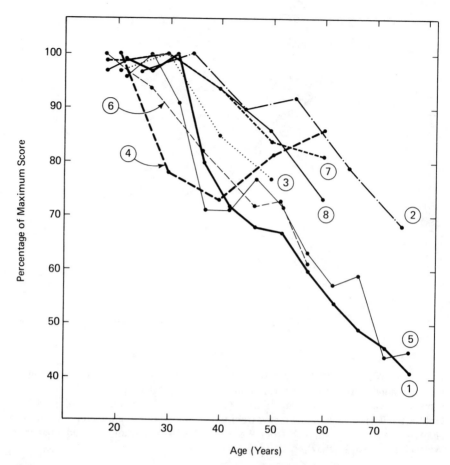

Figure 4.10. WAIS Block Design score at various ages expressed as a percentage of the maximum score across all ages. Numbers refer to different samples: 1 = adapted from Berkowitz (1953); 2 = adapted from Botwinick & Storandt (1974a); 3 = adapted from Goldfarb (1941)—females; 4 = adapted from Goldfarb (1941)—males; 5 = adapted from Howell (1955); 6 = adapted from Wechsler (1944); 7 = adapted from Wechsler (1958)—females; and 8 = adapted from Wechsler (1958)—males.

Nuttall, 1971; Glanzer et al. 1958; Helander, 1967; Heron & Chown, 1967; Heston & Cannell, 1941; Horn & Cattell, 1966, 1967; Kamin, 1957; Kennedy, 1981; Lee & Pollack, 1978; Mason & Ganzler, 1964; Muhs et al. 1979; Schaie et al. 1953; Schaie & Strother, 1968a, 1968b; Weisenburg et al. 1936; Westworth-Rohr, Mackintosh, & Fialkoff, 1974; Wilson et al. 1975).

Perceptual-Motor Speed

The WAIS Digit Symbol Substitution test is often considered to be a test that primarily emphasizes speed, although it has been suggested that spatial

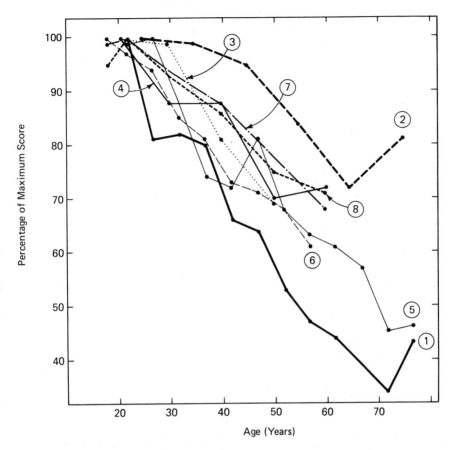

Figure 4.11. WAIS Picture Arrangement score at various ages expressed as a percentage of the maximum score across all ages. Numbers refer to different samples: 1 = adapted from Berkowitz (1953); 2 = adapted from Botwinick & Storandt (1974a); 3 = adapted from Goldfarb (1941)—females; 4 = adapted from Goldfarb (1941)—males; 5 = adapted from Howell (1955); 6 = adapted from Wechsler (1944); 7 = adapted from Wechsler (1958)—females; and 8 = adapted from Wechsler (1958)—males.

and memory factors also contribute to performance on this test. The examinee's task is to write the symbols associated with particular digits in boxes below the digits. The score is based on the number of correct digit-symbol substitutions completed in a 90-second period. Performance on this test as a function of age is displayed in Figure 4.12. It is obvious that there is substantial age-associated decline as the function indicates that performance decreases by a little more than 10% per decade. Slightly different substitution tests have also yielded very similar steep cross-sectional age declines (e.g., Heron & Chown, 1967; Weisenburg, Roe, & McBride, 1936; Willoughby, 1927), as have alternative psychometric measures of perceptual-motor speed (e.g., Bilash & Zubek, 1960; Schaie & Strother, 1968a).

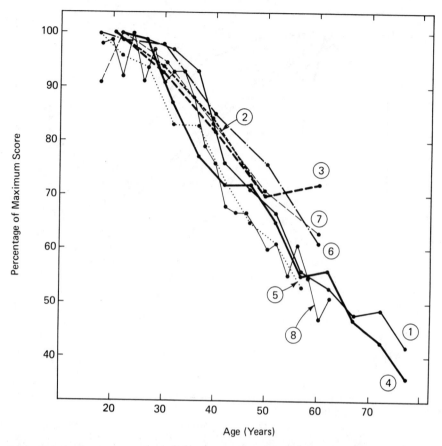

Figure 4.12. WAIS Digit Symbol score at various ages expressed as a percentage of the maximum score across all ages. Numbers refer to different samples: 1 = adapted from Berkowitz (1953); 2 = adapted from Goldfarb (1941)—females; 3 = adapted from Goldfarb (1941)—males; 4 = adapted from Howell (1955); 5 = adapted from Wechsler (1944); 6 = adapted from Wechsler (1958)—females; 7 = adapted from Wechsler (1958)—males; and 8 = adapted from Whiteman & Jastak (1957).

Reasoning Abilities

The WAIS has occasionally been criticized for not containing any measures of reasoning ability besides the Similarities test which is very dependent upon prior stored information. One type of reasoning test that is included in many other intelligence scales is the series completion test. The items in this test may be either letters or digits, but in either case the examinee is presented with a number of the items ordered in some sequence and the task is to supply the next item in the sequence. For example, a number completion problem might involve the presentation of the numbers 3-6-9 with the examinee instructed to provide the next number expected in the sequence. Performance on several tests of this type as a function of adult age is summarized in Figure

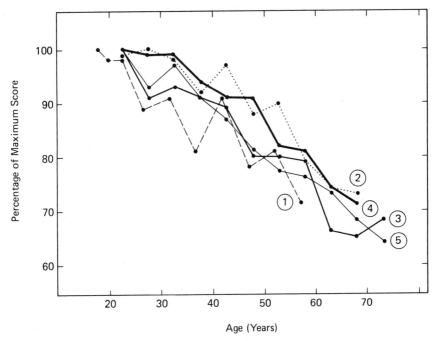

Figure 4.13. Series Completion reasoning score at various ages expressed as a percentage of the maximum score across all ages. Numbers refer to different samples: 1 = adapted from Jones & Conrad (1933); 2 = adapted from Schaie & Strother (1968a)—1956 males; 3 = adapted from Schaie & Strother (1968a)—1963 males; 4 = adapted from Schaie & Strother (1968a)—1956 females; 5 = adapted from Schaie & Strother (1968a)—1963 females.

4.13. As can be seen, reasoning performance exhibits cross-sectional declines of 6%–7% per decade beginning at about age 25 or 30. Similar results have been reported by Bilash and Zubek (1960) and Kamin (1957).

A second type of reasoning test involves nonverbal analogical reasoning in which the examinee is presented with three spatial patterns, and is required to select a fourth pattern that would possess the same relationship to the third pattern that the second pattern possesses with respect to the first. A very simple problem might contain a complete circle and a half circle as the first two patterns, and a complete square as the third pattern. In this case, the examinee should select a half square as the fourth pattern because it has the same half-to-complete relationship to the complete square as the half circle does to the complete circle. The best known test of this type is Raven's Progressive Matrices, and age functions for this test are illustrated in Figure 4.14. These data indicate that the cross-sectional age decline may not begin until about age 40, but once it starts the rate of loss is approximately 10% per decade. Similar age differences with this test have been reported by Chown (1961), Cunningham, Clayton, and Overton (1975), Davies and Leytham (1964), Davies, Spelman, and Davies (1981), Farrimond (1967), Foulds and

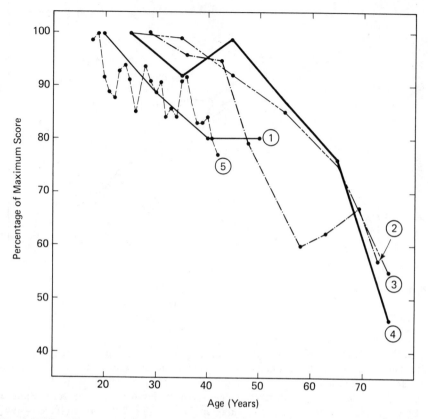

Figure 4.14. Raven's Progressive Matrices score at various ages expressed as a percentage of the maximum score across all ages. Numbers refer to different samples: 1 = adapted from Burke (1972); 2 = adapted from Edwards & Wine (1963); 3 = adapted from Heron & Chown (1967)—females; 4 = adapted from Heron & Chown (1967)—males; and 5 = adapted from Slater (1948).

Raven (1948), Guttman (1981), Mergler and Hoyer (1981), Muhs et al. (1979), Panek and Stoner (1980), Wilson et al. (1975) and Wilson (1963).

Characterizing the Differential Decline

The preceding sections have clearly indicated that the component abilities included in standardized tests of intelligence exhibit quite distinct developmental trends. Some abilities, such as previously acquired verbal skills, appear essentially invariant across most of the adult life span, but others, such as spatial abilities, begin to exhibit cross-sectional age differences as early as age 30 or 40. At the present time it is not known whether these different developmental trends are caused by variations in the proportion of reliance on a single mechanism, or by a number of separate mechanisms each with varying sensitivity to the effects of aging.

Although no generally accepted explanations for the differential declines are yet available, many descriptions of the differential decline pattern have been provided. Examples of several of the dichotomies suggested for characterizing the abilities that do, and do not, decline with age are listed in Table 4.1. In general, most of the descriptions suggest that increased age is associated with an impairment of ability to acquire or use new information. This characteristic is also one of the principal assumptions of a more elaborate descriptive system that makes a distinction between fluid and crystallized intelligence.

Horn (1967, 1970, 1975, 1978), Horn and Cattell (1966, 1967), and Horn and Donaldson (1976, 1977, 1980) have repeatedly suggested that developmental trends in intelligence can be understood in terms of a distinction between two major types of intelligence. One type, called fluid intelligence, is expected to decrease with increased age in adulthood. It is assumed to be reflected in tests of figural relations, memory span, induction, and most processes involved in acquiring new information. The second type of intelligence, called crystallized intelligence, is assumed to be the cumulative end product of information acquired by the activity of fluid intelligence processes. It is thus the sum total of the culturally dependent information stored by the individual as a result of his or her interactions in the environment. Crystallized

Table 4.1 Descriptions of Stable and Declining Abilities

Age Stable	Age Decline	Author
Accumulative effects of differential experience	Native capacity or "sheer modifiability"	Jones & Conrad (1933)
Language functions	Nonlanguage functions	Weisenburg et al. (1936)
Recall acquired information	Understand and adopt new methods of thinking	Foulds & Raven (1948)
Familiar materials	Abstract materials	Brown & Ghiselli (1949)
Accumulation of verbal or factual information	Flexible use of mental resources	Jones (1955)
Verbal abilities	Performance abilities	Wechsler (1958)
Stored information	Immediate adaptive ability	Reed & Reitan (1963)
Static intelligence	Flexible intelligence	Verhage (1965)
Specialized abilities	Unspecialized abilities	Bromley (1974)
Structure	Process	Kinsbourne (1974)
Utilization of stored information	Processing and integrating new information	Botwinick (1975)

intelligence is presumed to be measured by such tests as vocabulary, general information, comprehension, arithmetic, and reasoning with familiar material.

The fluid-crystallized dichotomy may or may not prove to be useful in describing the differential age trends in various intelligence subtests, but as it currently stands it represents no more of an explanation than any of the other descriptions listed in Table 4.1. The classification of a particular ability as fluid or crystallized seems to be somewhat arbitrary and based primarily on the observed developmental trend rather than a priori considerations. What is needed is some means of identifying the neurological processes responsible for a given ability such that the classification of abilities into fluid and crystallized groupings could be verified with neurological observations. Horn's (1975) speculation that fluid intelligence might be based on generalized, diffuse neural activity while crystallized intelligence is derivable from focused, specific neural activity is a step in this direction, but much more elaboration of mechanisms is necessary before the fluid-crystallized classification system can be considered a true theory of intellectual development.

Issues of Controversy

Does Intelligence Decline with Age?

It should be quite clear from the discussion thus far that different component abilities from intelligence tests exhibit quite different trends across the adult life span. It follows from this differential decline of subtests that the question of whether intelligence remains stable or declines depends upon the particular composite abilities included in the global test of intelligence. Based on the subtests discussed in the preceding sections, we could predict that scores on an intelligence test composed of Information, Vocabulary, and Comprehension subtests would be fairly stable across the adult life span, but scores on a test comprised of Digit Symbol, Picture Arrangement, and Object Assembly subtests would drop dramatically with increased age in cross-sectional samples. Global measures of intelligence are thus simply not suitable for analyzing adult changes in intellectual behavior because the nature of the function for the global measure is completely dependent upon the particular combination of subtests included in that intelligence scale. Moreover, in many cases the specific combination of subtests included in a global intelligence scale is rather arbitrary, although it is true that extensive validating studies have been carried out with most intelligence scales.

One implication of this argument is that the relationship between age and intellectual ability must be examined separately for each component ability. Neither comparisons of two different global tests, nor of the same global test at different ages, are meaningful if an identical total score can be achieved by various combinations of subtest scores. Abandoning the concept of global intelligence in favor of component abilities in discussions of adult development should therefore eliminate much of the confusion (and emotionality) associated with the utilization of the same term, intelligence, to refer to a large variety of behaviors.

Are Intelligence Tests Valid for Older Adults?

Another issue that is often raised concerning the age-intelligence relationship concerns the applicability of intelligence tests originally devised for children to the assessment of adults. The argument is that intelligence tests were constructed to predict success in academic environments, and although they have been relatively successful in that context, there is no comparable criterion with which to judge their success with adults who are no longer within academic settings. To some extent this argument is based on an assumption that academic intelligence, as measured by traditional intelligence tests, is not the same thing as "real-world intelligence." Unfortunately, there is not yet any satisfactory measure of this other type of intelligence.

Demming and Pressey (1957) attempted to provide a test that would sample practical, as opposed to academic, behaviors, and found that older adults were actually superior to most young adults on such a test. Their test was primarily a test of general information, however, and many would object to this measure of stored information as an index of intelligence. Moreover, other investigators have administered tests of information related to one's occupation and found slight but consistent cross-sectional age declines of the type reported with traditional intelligence tests (e.g., Glanzer & Glazer, 1959; Lefever, Van Boven, & Banarer, 1946). It has also been reported that there are sizable age differences in untimed tests of critical thinking ability involving problems related to daily experiences (e.g., Burton & Joel, 1945; Friend & Zubek, 1958), and in tests of ability to follow directions (e.g., Jones & Conrad, 1933; Price, 1933), and of "common sense" but not general information (e.g., Jones & Conrad, 1933). The consistency across these quite different tests suggests that the age-associated decline in intellectual abilities is real, and not merely a consequence of assessing intelligence with a contrived set of subtests originally invented for assessing children.

A reasonable conclusion with respect to the issue of whether intelligence tests are valid for older adults is that no conclusion can yet be reached. Largely because of the problem of defining an appropriate criterion for adult intelligence, the validity issue must still be considered an open question. One fact is clear, however, and that is that many of the component abilities used to measure intelligence, regardless of their respective validities in nonacademic contexts, do tend to have substantially lower scores with increased age. Therefore, to the extent that a valid test is developed in the future which relies on these component abilities, we can expect that it too will exhibit sizable cross-sectional age declines.

The Role of Speed

Many critics have claimed that the speeded nature of most intelligence tests unfairly penalizes older adults. The major assumption of this argument seems to be that speed loss is a peripheral, or extrinsic, factor that is irrelevant to the measurement of intelligence. Jones (1959) has summarized this position in the following query:

> We permit a 60-year-old man to wear his bifocals when he takes a mental test. Why should we not adjust the test to his changed speed requirements as well?" (1959, p. 722)

The problem with attempting to eliminate speed considerations from tests of intellectual ability is that, as Wechsler (1958) has pointed out, the older adult may not simply be slower, he or she may be "slowed-up." That is, the slower performance of older individuals may be a reflection of an intrinsic characteristic of the nervous system, and not merely a slowing of response or motor processes.

There are also several empirical arguments against removing speed considerations from intelligence tests. For example, it is generally found that speeded tests such as the WAIS Digit Symbol subtest correlate very highly with other nonspeeded subtests, suggesting that loss of speed is intrinsic to many intellectual processes. It has also been frequently reported that removing the time limits from a particular subtest does not alter the age relationships to any significant degree; older adults are still much less proficient than younger adults (e.g., Doppelt & Wallace, 1955; Gilbert, 1935; Klodin, 1976; C. Miles, 1934; Schaie et al. 1953; Storandt, 1977). Furthermore, Jones and Conrad (1933) have argued that the content of the test material is much more important than the presence of time limits as both the Information and Analogies subtests of the Army Alpha have time limits, but only in the Analogies subtest are substantial impairments evident in older individuals.

There can be no doubt that older adults are slower than young adults; however it does not seem legitimate to attempt to remove these effects in order to obtain "purer" estimates of intelligence. Salthouse (in press) has argued that the majority of the evidence indicates that age-related slowing is primarily a reflection of central nervous system deterioration. To the extent that slowing is centrally determined, removal of speed factors will tend to eliminate genuine effects of aging. Jones and Kaplan (1945) have also pointed out that there is no evidence that tests without time limits have any validity as tests of intelligence; they may merely reward patience and persistence instead of intellectual competence.

One additional point should be mentioned concerning the role of speed in tests of intelligence. Several investigators have claimed that the age relationship in a particular subtest can be changed by analyzing performance only with the first half of the test items rather than the entire test. A classic example of this outcome is a study by Christian and Paterson (1936) in which an age decline in the complete test was eliminated by considering performance only on the items from the first half of the test. The Christian and Paterson (1936) test involved vocabulary material and since nonspeeded tests indicate no age decline with such material the procedure may have been legitimate in their case. In other situations, however, this procedure may be inappropriate because many tests are constructed such that items become progressively more difficult in later sections of the test. Eliminating the last half of the test would therefore make the test easier, in addition to minimizing the role of speed. An investigator employing such a procedure should therefore be quite cautious in attributing any change in age relationships to the factor of speed rather than the factor of test difficulty.

The Role of Education

It has been noted earlier that intelligence tests were originally designed as a means of predicting academic success. If the tests are valid in this context, we would expect test performance to be highly correlated with educational achievement in quantitative, as well as qualitative, respects. In fact, correlations between test score and number of years of education in adults range from .40 to .66 across the WAIS subtests (Wechsler, 1958). On the average, the greater the number of years of schooling, the higher is the score. It is also known that adult age is negatively correlated with amount of education since educational opportunities have increased dramatically over the past 50 years or so.

Several investigators have argued that the positive correlation between amount of education and intelligence score, on the one hand, and the negative correlation between age and amount of education, on the other hand, may lead to a spurious age-related decrease in measured intelligence. In other words, the critical factor in the decline in measured intelligence may not be a deterioration associated with increased age, but instead an increase in quantity and quality of education in younger adults.

Several pieces of evidence have been presented in support of this line of reasoning. First, a number of large studies with the WAIS (e.g., Birren & Morrison, 1961; Granick & Friedman, 1967; Green, 1969) have demonstrated that many of the age differences in intellectual abilities are greatly reduced or even eliminated by matching individuals of various ages in terms of the number of years of education. And second, there have been reports that scores are higher with more recent administrations of a test to individuals of the same age, and it has been suggested that this time-lag improvement is primarily caused by improvements in education.

The clearest cases of a time-lag improvement are the comparison of the 1939 standardization of the Wechsler-Bellevue, the predecessor of the WAIS, with the 1955 standardization of the WAIS, and the comparison of World War II soldiers tested with the World War I Army Alpha test. Wechsler (1958) reported that scores in the 1955 revision of the WAIS were consistently higher than those from the initial 1939 testing, and he attributed a portion of this improvement to the increased educational opportunities from 1939 to 1955. Tuddenham (1948) reported that soldiers in World War II produced an average score on the Army Alpha that fell at the 83rd percentile of the distribution from World War I, and he too suggested that the increase in educational level in the general population was probably responsible for at least some of the improved test performance. A number of smaller-scale studies have also reported positive time-lag effects with higher scores in more recent test administrations (e.g., Cunningham & Birren, 1976; Owens, 1966; Schaie & Labouvie-Vief, 1974; Schaie & Strother, 1968a), although at least two studies have failed to report substantial time-lag differences (e.g., Campbell, 1965; Garrison, 1930). While there does appear to be a trend for intellectual performance to be higher on more recent test administrations (at least over periods of decades rather than the last several years), educational opportunities are only one of many changes that occurred during the intervening interval and any of these progressive aspects may be responsible for the improved performance.

In interpreting the role of educational level on intelligence it is important to distinguish between amount of education as a cause, or as an effect, of level of intelligence. The mere presence of a correlation between the two variables is not informative about which variable is primarily responsible for the other. It seems reasonable to argue that intelligence is in some sense the "cause" of amount of education since each successive level of education presumably requires a higher minimum amount of intelligence. In order for the education contamination argument to have validity with respect to age-intelligence relationships, however, it must be assumed that an increase in years of education somehow "causes" an increase in intelligence. Although some educators might be willing to accept this particular direction in the relationship, there appears to be little evidence that merely increasing the amount of schooling substantially affects an individual's intellectual capacity. It is possible that increased educational experience alters an individual's interests or attitudes such that he or she maintains or even increases certain abilities across the life span instead of having them deteriorate, but it seems unlikely that the educational process itself is responsible for substantial increases in basic intellectual abilities.

Another objection to the education artifact interpretation is that making individuals of various age groups equivalent in terms of the number of years of education does not match them in terms of quality of education, or in the number of years since schooling. With the increase in the average number of years of education there has also been a dramatic change in the qualitative nature of instruction. The educational facilities, the extensiveness of the teachers' training and preparation, and even the dominant mode of instruction, i.e., rote versus discovery, have all changed over the past 50 years and it may be unrealistic to assume that a year of education has had the same impact on the individual at all periods in our history. Furthermore, it is generally impossible to balance the number of years since the formal educational experience, and cumulative forgetting would appear to impair the performance of the older individual more than the younger one. That is, if specific information acquired during the periods of formal education is assumed to be important in influencing intelligence scores, then the older adult is at a disadvantage with respect to the younger adult because of the greater time that has elapsed in which forgetting may be taking place. The net effect of these considerations is difficult to estimate, but it does appear that the strategy of matching individuals of different ages on the basis of years of education is rather naive, and the results of such a procedure do not lend themselves to simple interpretations.

A related objection was briefly mentioned in Chapter 2. This concerns the comparability of individuals in different ages who are matched on years of education when the educational trends have changed so dramatically in recent history. A college graduate in the 1930s was a member of a relatively small, and elite, minority among his or her age cohorts, whereas a much larger proportion of young people are graduating from college in the 1980s. The mere fact that an individual was attending college in the 1930s signified that his or her family was probably well-to-do and highly educated, but college attendance in the 1980s is less informative about the family's socioeconomic status. Since college attendance was more highly related to socioeconomic status in previous years than at the present time, and since socioeconomic status has been found to be related to intelligence, it might be argued that older college graduates were initially more intelligent, on the average, than young college graduates. This argument implies that matching on the basis of education to examine intelligence may be actually contaminating the age differences by means of biasing the various age samples.

There is also an empirical argument against the education artifact explanation of the age-intelligence relationship. If educational differences are partially responsible for the observed age differences in intellectual abilities, one would expect the age differences to be greatest on those subtests that are most similar to the type of material studied in school. However, many years ago Jones and Conrad (1933) and Willoughby (1927) pointed out that the most dramatic age differences were in subtests such as the series completion, analogies, and digit symbol substitution, which are quite dissimilar to school-trained information. The subtests that did involve material related to school, e.g., vocabulary, general information, and arithmetic, were found not to decline with increased age. This general trend is also evident in the WAIS subtests discussed earlier, and seems to argue against the hypothesis that educational differences are major contributors to the age-related decline in measured intelligence.

Cross-Sectional versus Longitudinal Results

It has sometimes been suggested that longitudinal studies of intellectual ability portray a very different developmental trend from cross-sectional studies, and that the results from cross-sectional studies might therefore be misleading if considered in isolation. Actually, one of the first longitudinal studies of intelligence, i.e., C. Miles (1934), reported that the longitudinal decrease over a two-year period in the same individuals was very similar to the cross-sectional decrease over a comparable age span for individuals of different ages. In other words, this initial study indicated that longitudinal and cross-sectional designs produced nearly identical results. More recent studies, however, have revealed that longitudinal age differences in intellectual functions are often considerably smaller than those reported in cross-sectional studies. The best known example of this discrepancy comes from a comparison of the Jones and Conrad (1933) cross-sectional study and the Owens (1953) longitudinal study, both using the Army Alpha test. Unlike Jones and Conrad, Owens found that college-educated adults changed very little, or even improved, on the Army Alpha over a 25-year span. Several other studies have also been reported in which the longitudinal age differences were much smaller than might be expected on the basis of cross-sectional results (e.g., Bayley & Owen, 1955; Glanzer & Glazer, 1959; Kangas & Bradway, 1971; Nisbet, 1957; Schaie & Labouvie-Vief, 1974; Schaie & Strother, 1968a; Tuddenham, Blumenkrantz, & Wilkin, 1968).

Although many researchers have been impressed with these apparent differences, the discrepancies in results with cross-sectional and longitudinal designs seem to be explainable if one considers the particular measures of intelligence employed, the age span investigated, and the problems of sampling bias inherent in longitudinal studies (e.g., Botwinick, 1977; Horn & Donaldson, 1976, 1980). As an example, several of the studies cited above (e.g., Bayley & Owen, 1955; Nisbet, 1957) employed tests primarily assessing verbal ability as the measure of intelligence, and it has been noted earlier that verbal ability remains fairly stable across the life span with the tests currently available. The absence of a decline with such tests of intelligence is thus consistent with what would occur in a cross-sectional study employing a similar verbal ability test.

Most of the longitudinal studies have also been severely restricted in the span of ages involved. For instance, Bayley and Owen (1955) compared individuals at ages 30 and 42, Nisbet (1957) compared individuals at ages 23 and 47, and Kangas and Bradway (1971) contrasted 30-year-olds with 44-year-olds. This is a segment of the age span in which the decline may not be particularly prominent as the peak years in the early 20s are not included, and the later years where the decline is most evident are also absent.

One of the most important factors involved in the apparent discrepancy between cross-sectional and longitudinal results is the selective attrition operating in nearly all of the available longitudinal studies. C. Miles (1934), in one of the first longitudinal studies, noted that there was actually a gain in the scores of individuals who readily volunteered for retesting, but that inclusion of the more reluctant participants from the initial testing led to an overall decline in test score. Such a retest bias, with the least competent individuals being less available for retesting, has probably been contributing to the results of most longitudinal studies. Since this selective attrition is progressive, the overall effect would be a distorted age relationship with the older ages much more favorably represented than the younger ages. Excellent discussions of how such selective attrition can affect the results and interpretations from the longitudinal data of Schaie and his colleagues (e.g., Schaie & Labouvie-Vief, 1974; Schaie & Strother, 1968a) have recently been presented by Botwinick (1977) and Horn and Donaldson (1976, 1980).

While Schaie and his colleagues have argued that nonmaturational factors are responsible for many of the age differences typically reported with psychometric measures of intelligence, one is struck by the remarkably similar age trends in his data from different measurement periods. Nearly identical age trends are evident in the cross-sectional comparisons from the 1956, 1963, and 1970 measurement periods (e.g., Schaie & Labouvie-Vief, 1974; Schaie & Strother, 1968a) for almost all intellectual variables. For several of the variables the absolute level of performance changed across successive measurement periods, thus causing the longitudinal results to exhibit slightly different age trends than the cross-sectional results. However, both the direction and the magnitude of the change over successive measurement periods varied across dependent variables and thus the effect is not yet systematic enough to allow specification of its exact nature.

With the exception of the sizable time-of-measurement effects, Schaie's cross-sectional data portray a pattern of age trends very similar to those described earlier in this chapter, although perhaps with somewhat more dramatic age differences in the measure of vocabulary (verbal meaning) than generally found. Schaie's longitudinal data indicate a slightly more gradual aging trend, but do not differ qualitatively from his cross-sectional findings.

In view of the preceding arguments it seems reasonable to conclude that the discrepancy between longitudinal and cross-sectional studies is more apparent than real. Kuhlen's (1963) observation that the longitudinal data are too tenuous to allow definitive statements about the relationship between the two types of data collection is still valid, but the presently available evidence is not particularly compelling concerning the hypothesis that there is a fundamentally different pattern of results on adult intelligence with the two methods.

Miscellaneous Extraneous Factors

In addition to the major issues discussed above, a number of other factors have been proposed as being responsible for reducing the older individual's performance below his or her actual level of competence. Because these factors are assumed to be extrinsic to the individual's true ability or competence, they are considered to be extraneous to the measurement of real intelligence.

One such extraneous factor is motivational level. It has occasionally been suggested that older adults perform poorly on experimental and psychometric tasks because they are less motivated in those activities than young adults. Although this argument has intuitive plausibility (particularly when one compares older adults to college students who seem willing and even enthusiastic to perform the most trivial and mundane activities under the guise of psychological experiments), there is apparently no empirical evidence to support such a speculation. Indeed, when only highly motivated individuals are tested (e.g., Ganzler, 1964; Schaie & Strother, 1968b), the age differences are of about the same magnitude as those reported in other studies. Also, Jones and Kaplan (1945) have noted that reduced motivation is most likely to be manifested in refusal to participate in the research project, and yet when individuals who initially refuse are finally coerced into participating, the cross-sectional age declines are often greater than those reported in the initial sample (e.g., Jones & Conrad, 1933).

Judging from some of the statements concerning the role of motivation, there appears to be considerable confusion about the relationship between motivation and ability. One of the clearest statements of this relationship was made by Jones:

> We sometimes speak of motivation as though it were a prime mover which could be turned on or off irrespective of target mechanisms. But motivation and ability are usually interactive. We like to do things that we can do well. We become resistant toward activities which reveal our shortcomings. (1959, p. 718)

To state that older adults do not perform well on activities for which they have not been reinforced recently is therefore not an explanation. What is necessary is a determination of whether the reinforcements were lacking because the performance was inferior, or the performance was inferior because the reinforcements were lacking. This is an empirical issue that must ultimately be resolved with data, and cannot simply be dismissed with emotional appeals.

Three other factors that have been discussed as performance-limiting extraneous factors working against older adults are practice, fatigue, and cautiousness. Several studies have been reported in which some type of intervention program was implemented to remedy the lack of practice, greater susceptibility to fatigue, or excessive cautiousness suspected to be limiting the performance of older adults in assessment situations. For example, Hoyer, Labouvie, and Baltes (1973), Kamin (1957), and Plemons, Willis, and Baltes (1978) administered practice treatments; Cunningham, Sepkoski, and Opel (1978), Furry and Baltes (1973), Hayslip and Sterns (1979), and Kamin (1957) investigated fatigue manipulations; and Birkhill and Schaie (1975) studied the effects of a treatment designed to reduce excessive cautiousness. Unfortunately, many of these studies did not include a young control group and, as Horn and Donaldson (1976) pointed out, without such an age comparison the studies simply do not address the age difference issue. The outcome of studies with only one age group contribute very little to an understanding of why one age group is different from another. Furthermore, in the studies that did include at least two different age groups, only Furry and Baltes (1973) reported a significant age by treatment (fatigue) interaction, and this was not confirmed by Cunningham et al. (1978), Hayslip and Sterns (1979) or Kamin (1957). Without clear evidence of a differential effect of the treatment such that one age group benefits more than another, it is impossible to claim that any of these extraneous factors contributes to the differences observed between various age groups.

Another extraneous factor that has been mentioned as influencing the performance of older adults is auditory sensitivity. Granick, Kleban, and Weiss (1976) reported that many of the subtests of the WAIS are moderately correlated with degree of hearing loss such that the greater the hearing impairment, the poorer the performance on the subtest. While suggestive, these results should be interpreted with considerable caution. The particular subtests that exhibited high correlations (e.g., the digit symbol substitution test) were not related to auditory sensitivity in any intuitively obvious manner, while other tests that might be expected to be related did not have high correlations (e.g., the digit span test). Further, in order to claim that the age differences are at least partially attributable to differences in auditory sensitivity, it would have been desirable to demonstrate that a group of young adults with comparable auditory impairments produced similar decrements in performance. Only older adults were included in the Granick et al. (1976) study, and thus the significance of the correlations to the question of the cause of age differences in intellectual performance could not be assessed.

Individual Differences

A point that deserves special emphasis when considering the topic of intelligence is that there are tremendous individual differences in the rate of change in intellectual abilities, just as there are very large differences in the peak levels of these abilities. In fact, the correlations between chronological age and raw scores on subtests of intelligence seldom exceed .5, which although often considered sizable, indicates that only about 25% of the variability in intelligence scores can be accounted for by knowledge of age. The results discussed in this chapter have referred to statistical averages, and therefore they are of very little use in attempting to predict the performance of a specific individual.

There have been some reports that the rate of decline in intelligence is less rapid in the initially more intelligent individuals (e.g., Blum & Jarvik, 1974; Foulds & Raven, 1948; Gilbert, 1935; Riegel & Riegel, 1972; Shakow & Goldman, 1938), but Baltes, Nesselroade, Schaie, and Labouvie (1972) have presented a convincing argument that many of these results might be explainable by a statistical regression artifact. (These authors employed an intriguing time-reversed analysis procedure in which forward, i.e., 1956–1963, and backward, i.e., 1963–1956, comparisons were examined.) At the present time, then, it is probably not wise to draw any conclusions about differential rates of declines across particular groups of individuals. It is obvious that people vary greatly in their specific patterns of aging; it is just not possible at the current time to characterize the commonalities responsible for particular aging trends.

Theoretical Evaluation

In view of the evidence that the various component abilities in intelligence tests exhibit substantially different developmental trends, any theoretical discussion of intelligence must be rather vague. Intelligence is a multifaceted concept, particularly when viewed from an adult development perspective, and thus it is impossible to be very concrete in one's theoretical speculations. Nevertheless, it is still worthwhile to examine some of the major theoretical issues from the context of the literature surveyed in this chapter.

With respect to theories stressing a biological (maturational) determinant of age changes, three observations may be considered as favorable evidence. The first is that the intellectual ability decline associated with increased age has at least a superficial similarity to the impairments associated with diffuse brain damage (e.g., Davies, 1968; Davies et al. 1981; Reed & Reitan, 1963; but see Overall & Gorham, 1972), suggesting that organic factors might be responsible for the aging deficits. Second, the decline with most abilities is more continuous than abrupt, and thus seems characteristic of a gradual biological process. An environmental determinant of the observed aging differences might be expected to be more abrupt as an individual suddenly retires and is removed from previous reinforcements or stimulation. And third, there is some indication that the age decline is greatest on tests that are most unfamiliar and least dependent upon specific experience, e.g., the spatial abilities tests and the digit symbol substitution test. Since these tests are unlikely to have been "contaminated" by social or cultural factors, they might be interpreted as providing the best index of the biological deterioration that underlies all mental performance.

Environmentally oriented theories of age differences can also claim support from the literature on adult intelligence. Many researchers have argued that increased age is associated with a progressively narrower range of interests and activities such that certain activities can no longer be performed as well because they are less often practiced (e.g., Granick & Friedman, 1967; Heron & Chown, 1967; Jones & Conrad, 1933; Schaie et al. 1953; Sorenson, 1938; Tuddenham et al. 1968; Williams, 1960). It has also been pointed out that abilities that are in continuous use throughout the life span, such as vocabulary and other verbal abilities in teachers (e.g., Garfield & Blek, 1952; Nisbet, 1957; Sorenson, 1933; Sward, 1945), either do not decline, or possibly even increase, with increased age. On the other hand, attempts to relate the rate of decline on particular tests to the type of activity in which the individual has been engaged in the years intervening between successive testings have not revealed any significant relationships (e.g., Green & Reimanis, 1970; Owens, 1953; but see Kohn & Schooler, 1978 for an interesting exception). It should also be noted that Kamin (1957) found that older adults did not improve any more than young adults when provided with practice, i.e., given additional administrations of the same test.

The competence-performance distinction has been the subject of considerable speculation within the field of adult intelligence, but as yet there is little solid evidence in either direction. Some researchers have argued that age-associated performance declines are not accurate reflections of true competence, and consequently have examined a number of manipulations designed to optimize performance of older adults. Unfortunately, most of these studies failed to include a young adult group and thus it cannot be determined whether performance below the level of one's competence is unique to older adults. It is clear that much more research, with at least two age groups, is needed in this area. At the current time there simply is not enough data to justify any conclusion on the competence-performance issue.

In view of the widely varying developmental trends for different component abilities, it seems likely that successful theories in this area must be specific rather than general. Only if it is eventually determined that the assorted abilities all depend, in varying proportions, upon a single mechanism or process would a general theory appear credible.

To summarize, the presently available literature in psychometric intelligence does not allow strong conclusions about theoretical issues. There is mixed evidence concerning maturational versus environmental determinants of the observed results, and no useful evidence concerning the performance versus competence distinction. The most that can be said is that it is unlikely that a single general theory will be able to account for the diverse age trends observed across the domains of ability typically included in tests of intelligence.

Summary

Although nearly every other conceivable issue seems to have been debated, the fundamental fact that intelligence as assessed by traditional intelligence tests with cross-sectional procedures exhibits more or less continuous decreases across successive age groups beginning at about age 25–30 has not been disputed. Many psychologists, like Spearman (1927), have been impressed by the "tragical import" of this finding and have speculated that humans are already too old for their best work at age 30, rather than 50 or 70. Wechsler (1958) and others, however, have noted that intelligence is not the only factor involved in human accomplishments, and that wisdom, judgment, and sagacity are dependent more on actual experience than sheer capacity. It is likely that knowledge acquired through experience is often as important as intelligence in human activities, and experience is generally to the advantage of the older individual.

It is also important to note that the decline is continuous rather than abrupt and thus the loss of intellectual ability may be as important a consideration in a comparison of 50-year-olds with 30-year-olds, as it is in a comparison of 70-year-olds with 50-year-olds. The important question in many evaluations of adults seems to be whether the individual can handle the tasks of interest, rather than the position on the decline function. Since most abilities exhibit gradual decline, such that even at age 70 there is considerable residual ability that may be sufficient for the performance of many activities, data of the type discussed in this chapter may be quite useless for most predictive purposes.

One of the major assertions in this chapter was that intelligence is not a single, unitary trait (at least with respect to how it is measured), but instead consists of a combination of developmentally distinct component abilities. The implication of this view is that it does not make sense to attempt to examine the relationship between age and a unidimensional index of global intelligence. Each of the component abilities must be examined separately if any understanding of causal factors is to be obtained. Such a detailed examination is conducted in the following chapters as the focus shifts from a psychometric perspective, in which the concern was with descriptive information about relative ability, to an experimental perspective, in which the mechanisms and processes responsible for particular levels of performance are analyzed.

5. Decision Making and Problem Solving

Imagine that you have been placed in the position of screening applicants for a high-level decision-making position. What criteria would you employ to evaluate the candidates for a job that involves making important decisions and solving difficult problems? Perhaps the first attribute that you would look for would be previous experience in making similar types of decisions or solving related problems. It is reasonable to expect that someone who has enjoyed success in such situations in the past will likely prove successful in the future. However, if experience is excluded, other characteristics must be considered. Some of those that might be useful in this context are: (1) creativity; (2) flexibility; (3) organizational skills; (4) ability to make valid logical deductions; (5) ability to sift relevant from irrelevant information; (6) ability to operate at both abstract and concrete levels; and (7) ability to proceed systematically towards a problem solution.

Although the amount of research concerned with adult age and decision making or problem solving is not large, it is somewhat discouraging that age decrements have been reported in all the decision-making characteristics noted above. It is not possible to conclude on the basis of these findings that older adults are generally poorer decision makers than young adults because the contribution of sheer experience is unknown in most decision contexts, and undoubtedly of major importance. Nonetheless, the available evidence seems to portray a rather pessimistic view of the older adult as a decision maker in novel situations. In the present chapter we will examine this evidence to determine whether it is actually reasonable to conclude that there are substantial declines in "pure" decision-making abilities, independent of experience, as one grows older. Our coverage of the literature will be organized primarily in terms of the seven optimal decision-maker characteristics listed above.

Creativity

While creativity is one of the most valued attributes an individual could possess in modern society, it is unfortunately the case that there are very few accepted assessment techniques for the measurement of creativity. One fairly typical procedure simply asks individuals to name as many different uses as possible for a common object like a brick. The reasoning is that a great number of people will be able to provide a few familiar answers such as using it as a component in construction, but only the most creative people will be able to offer unique responses such as using the brick as a doorstop. The argument that unusual or infrequent responses are creative has some intuitive appeal, but we do not yet know whether these types of measures are really valid reflections of creativity as the term is commonly used. In the absence of any better assessment devices, however, the current tests of creativity will have to suffice if one wishes to make any statements about differences in creativity across groups of people.

Two slightly different types of tests have been employed in studies of the influence of aging on creativity, but both have used the "unique response" rationale just discussed. The Vygotsky Test consists of 22 wooden blocks in a variety of colors, shapes, heights, and widths. The task is to discover as many different sortings or arrangements of the blocks as possible. The Shaw Test is very similar but there are only four different blocks with a smaller number of dimensions of difference.

Bromley (1967) administered both the Shaw and Vygotsky Tests without time limits to 250 adults in three age groups with approximate age means of 27, 47, and 67 years. The mean number of responses in each test declined with increased age such that the individuals with a mean age of 67 years produced only 50%–66% as many different responses as the individuals with a mean age of 27 years (see Figure 5.1). This result is particularly impressive when it is noted that the participants in Bromley's study were all intellectually superior adults with approximately the same mean Wechsler-Bellevue Intelligence Score (i.e., means of 122 for the young adults, 123 for the middle-aged adults, and 121 for the older adults).

Bromley's interpretation of these results was that there is a decline in either persistence, flexibility, or abstraction—the combination of which is presumed to be necessary for a high score. Regardless of which specific process is primarily responsible, the results portrayed in Figure 5.1 clearly suggest that increased age is associated with a reduction in creativity, as measured by the number of different responses, even when the mean level of intelligence is held constant.

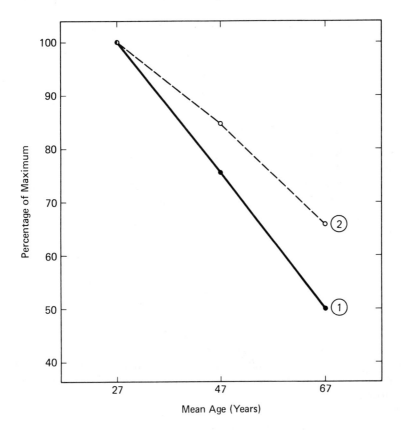

Figure 5.1. Shaw Test (1) and Vygotsky Test (2) scores at various ages expressed as a percentage of the maximum score across all ages. Data from Bromley (1967).

Alpaugh and Birren (1977) reported a striking confirmation of Bromley's results in a comparison of 111 adults between the ages of 20 and 83. Increased age was associated with poorer performance in a composite measure of creativity or divergent thinking, despite comparable levels of verbal intelligence across age groups.

Less dramatic age trends in creativity were reported in a recent study by Jaquish and Ripple (1981). However, the task employed in this study was very unstructured, with participants merely requested "to be imaginative" in writing reactions to auditory stimuli. Given such a vague task, it is not clear that the responses should be considered reflections of creativity rather than, for example, some dimension of personality. This latter interpretation is supported in the finding that the measures of "divergent thinking" reported by Jaquish and Ripple were significantly correlated with an index of self-esteem.

A test specifically designed to measure ingenuity was administered to 64 pilots by Glanzer et al. (1958). On the assumption that "an 'ingenious' person is one who can form relationships between things or ideas which are not generally thought of as one concept," pairs of words or pictures were presented with instructions to specify a relationship between the pair of items. A higher score on this "finding relations" test can therefore be interpreted as a reflection of greater creativity or ingenuity. Although no individuals over the age of 50 were tested, the correlation between adult age and this measure of creativity was $-.28$ ($p < .05$), indicating fewer ingenious or creative responses with increased age.

It would be very desirable to obtain additional evidence from other types of tests assessing creativity before drawing a firm conclusion, but at the present time the consistent results with relatively large samples in the Bromley (1967), Alpaugh and Birren (1977) and Glanzer et al. (1958) studies suggests that creativity, at least insofar as we can measure it in the laboratory, seems to be lower with increased age.

Flexibility

Flexibility is a desirable characteristic for a decision maker to the extent that it enables one to change his or her opinion in the face of new information. An inflexible or rigid individual would have a difficult time adapting to new situations and might even find it impossible to function under rapidly changing conditions.

Flexibility, or its converse, rigidity, has been measured in several ways. As was the case with creativity, however, the validity of the various measures is still not known. Each has a certain amount of face validity in that it seems to reflect ability or willingness to change, but large-scale empirical studies documenting the relationship between these measures and extralaboratory behaviors have not yet been reported.

One procedure to determine an individual's relative position on the flexibility-rigidity dimension requires the person to perform different operations either separately or in alternation, with the score being some comparison of the relative performance in the two conditions. For example, Botwinick, Brinley, and Robbin (1958) presented addition and subtraction problems separately or alternately, Schaie (1958) presented separate or alternating synonym and antonym questions, and Brinley (1965) presented both arithmetic and verbal items in this type of separate or alternating arrangement. The assumption is that an individual who requires more time when performing two operations in rapid alternation, compared to performing first one operation and then another, is less flexible than an individual whose performance is the same under separate and alternating conditions. The additional time required for the alternation of activity, independent of the activity time itself, is thus taken as an index of the individual's rigidity, or lack of flexibility.

Using this type of measure, all three of the studies cited above reported

Table 5.1 Motor-Cognitive Rigidity Measures Across the Adult Life Span

	Age									
	20-25	26-30	31-35	36-40	41-45	46-50	51-55	56-60	61-65	66-70
Percent of Maximum Score	100	95	96	88	90	91	86	82	80	73

Note. Adapted from Schaie & Strother, 1968a.

greater rigidity in older adults than in younger adults. Schaie's (1958) results, with 25 males and 25 females in each of ten 5-year age ranges, are displayed in Table 5.1. Notice that the age function, while not steep, exhibits a gradual reduction in flexibility, i.e., an increase in rigidity, with increasing age. This result, in conjunction with the similar findings by Botwinick et al. (1958) and Brinley (1965), strongly suggests that the ability to shift rapidly from one type of activity to another tends to decrease with increased age.

A second method of measuring an individual's position on the rigidity-flexibility dimension utilizes what has come to be known as the Einstellung procedure. Several different tasks have been used to investigate the Einstellung effect (e.g., the water-jug task, the alphabet-maze task, and the anagram task), but each follows the same basic logic. First, a series of problems is presented which can be solved only by a rather complicated solution. Later, several problems are introduced which can be solved with either the complicated solution or with a much simpler solution. And finally, one or more problems are presented in which only the simple solution is effective. The measure of rigidity or flexibility available from this procedure is the relative difficulty of solving the last problem. If an individual tends to persevere in a previously successful strategy that is no longer applicable, he or she will experience great difficulty with the final, new-solution, problem. On the other hand, if the person is flexible and readily adopts alternative strategies when the previous strategy is discovered to be ineffective, the final problem should not be excessively difficult.

The major aging study employing the Einstellung procedure was reported by Heglin (1956). One-hundred and fifty males and 150 females were administered the water-jug and alphabet-maze versions of the Einstellung task. The participants were divided into three age ranges, with 100 teenagers (age range 14–18, median age of 16), 100 young adults (age range 20–49, median age of 32), and 100 older adults (age range 50–85, median age of 66). Older adults were reported to experience more difficulty on the new-solution problems than the young adults on both the water-jug and alphabet-maze tasks. Older adults also benefited less than young adults from specific instructions warning about the tendency to use only one solution strategy for all problems. (The teenagers were either at the level of the young adults, or between the two adult groups, on all measures.)

Heglin's findings can be interpreted as indicating that older adults are less flexible than young adults in considering alternative solutions to a problem when the old solution no longer works. Our confidence in this conclusion should not be too great, however, since all of the results upon which it is based are derived from a single experiment.

A third measure that has been used as a reflection of rigidity or flexibility is obtained in concept-identification tasks. Typically a number of stimulus items for which one concept is "correct" are presented, and then either with or without the individual's awareness a new concept is substituted for the old one. For example, the stimuli might be cards that vary in the number, shape, color, and size of objects drawn upon them, with the individual instructed to determine which dimension or combination of dimensions is reponsible for some stimuli being classified positive and others negative. Initially the concept might be "red and square" such that any card with one or more red squares on it would be classified as positive and all other cards classified as negative. At the time of the transfer the concept might be shifted to some other set of dimensions (e.g., "two and large"), or to different values along the same dimensions (e.g., "blue and circular"). The relative difficulty of acquiring this new concept can be considered a measure of the individual's rigidity. A person low in rigidity, one who adapts easily to changes in the rules or requirements, would presumably not experience much difficulty in acquiring the new concept, whereas a highly rigid person might be expected to experience great difficulty and frustration when the "correct" concept is changed in the middle of an experiment.

Two studies have reported that young adults are more successful at shifting to a new concept than older adults, but each has some problems that limit the conclusions that can be drawn. Wetherick (1965) employed very few individuals in each age group and conducted no formal statistical analyses to evaluate the differences that were observed. Nehrke (1973) examined a larger number of participants, a total of 192 different individuals, but substantial age differences in the acquisition of the initial concept made it difficult to interpret the results with the changed concept. In light of these difficulties it is perhaps best to reserve judgment on whether this particular measure of rigidity exhibits sizable age differences.

It seems fairly certain that some aspects of flexibility tend to decline with increased age. The task-alternation and Einstellung procedures have yielded consistent results indicating lower levels of flexibility among older adults compared to young or middle-aged adults, and the available evidence on shifting concepts, although flawed, is also consistent with this conclusion.

Organizational Skills

An ideal decision maker or problem solver should possess the ability to organize seemingly unrelated aspects of a problem into a single, meaningful pattern. Many times the key to a problem solution lies in the manner in which it is organized; the right organization can make the solution trivial, and an inappropriate organization can make the problem nearly impossible.

Organizational abilities have been investigated in the laboratory by asking people to classify groups of stimulus items and examining either the number, or types, of groupings. The Shaw and Vygotsky Tests discussed earlier can therefore be interpreted as providing measures of organization. It will be remembered that Bromley (1967) found fewer different organizations of the stimulus items in the older age groups than in the young age groups. This result may indicate an organizational deficiency, in addition to a lower level of creativity, among elderly adults.

Two more recent studies, by Kogan (1974) and Cicirelli (1976), examined age differences in both the number and the type of groupings. As would be expected from Bromley's results, both investigators found that the older adults formed fewer groups than the young adults. However, it was also found in both studies that older adults tended to make proportionally more groupings on the basis of functional relationships among items than the young adults. For instance, a drawing of a stove and a drawing of a frying pan might be grouped together because the frying pan is used on the stove. A more abstract level of classification, exhibited with greater frequency by young adults, would involve the grouping of items by category. As an example, the drawing of the frying pan might be grouped with drawings of a tea kettle or a pot, while the drawing of the stove might be grouped with a drawing of a refrigerator or a dishwasher.

The difference in types of groupings does not necessarily mean that the older adults were completely defective in organizational skills, but it does suggest that the organizations formed by older adults relative to those formed by young adults are more often dominated by rather primitive relationships among items than by higher abstract categories. In this respect, therefore, the Kogan and Cicirelli results might be interpreted as indicating a weakness in certain types of organizational abilities in later adulthood. Experiments by Annett (1959) and Denney and Lennon (1972) also reported adult age differences in classification criteria and are thus consistent with the results and conclusions from the Kogan and Cicirelli studies.

A second technique that has been used in the laboratory to investigate organizational skills utilizes a variant of the familiar 20-questions game. In the version employed by Denney and her colleagues (e.g., Denney, 1980; Denney & Denney, 1973, 1982; Denney & Palmer, 1981; Kesler, Denney, & Whitely, 1976), the participants were presented with 42 pictures and instructed to ask questions to determine which picture the experimenter had designated as the target picture. Organization is important in this task to provide an initial grouping of the alternatives so that each question might serve to eliminate as many alternatives as possible. That is, grouping the pictures into, for example, animals and nonanimals, would allow a question about whether the target is an animal to eliminate many possibilities with a single question. This type of organization can be inferred by the proportion of total questions that are constraining in the sense of eliminating more than one alternative at

Table 5.2 Percentage of Constraining Questions in the 20-Questions Task

	Age					
	20-29	30-39	40-49	50-59	60-69	70-79
Percent of maximum score, Denney & Palmer (1981)	87	100	83	77	53	27
Percent of maximum score, Denney & Denney (1982)	—	100	92	74	58	44

a time. In all of the studies cited (i.e., Denney, 1980; Denney & Denney, 1973, 1982; Denney & Palmer, 1981; Kesler et al. 1976) it was reported that elderly adults (ages 65–81 years) required more questions to solution, and asked a smaller proportion of constraining questions, than did middle-aged adults (ages 30–50 years). Data for the percentage of constraining questions across the adult life span are illustrated in Table 5.2, although Denney and Palmer (1981) state that the value for the 30- to 39-year old group in their experiment is atypically high relative to other studies. Arenberg (1974), using a quite different experimental task, also reported an age-related increase in the number of uninformative questions, again suggesting a less effective problem organization among older adults.

Although one might have reservations about the validity of these laboratory measures of organizational ability, particularly if one is concerned with generalizing to complicated decision situations, it must be admitted that the results available thus far are reasonably consistent. Older adults apparently make fewer and less abstract organizations than younger adults, and also tend to rely less on self-generated organizations when seeking solutions to simple problems.

Ability to Make Logical Deductions

Logical consistency, both in drawing one's own conclusions and in evaluating the arguments of others, would seem to be a very desirable trait for a high-level decision maker. Many problem-solving situations involve inferences that go beyond the strict rules of logic, and yet it is inconceivable that one would be respected as a decision maker if he or she was unable to use deductive logic to identify the implications of an argument.

The most commonly used laboratory technique for investigating logical deductive ability involves some variant of a concept-identification task. Stimuli in concept-identification tasks are composed of several elements or dimensions, one (or a combination of two or more) of which is designated as defining the concept. The stimulus complexes are typically presented sequentially, with feedback provided about the concept identity after the individual's response. A concept is considered identified if the person can state the critical element or dimension, or can demonstrate this knowledge by performing for a certain number of trials without any errors.

Most concept-identification tasks have employed abstract stimulus dimensions such as color, shape, or size. However, Arenberg (1968a), and later Hayslip and Sterns (1979) and Hartley (1981), cleverly incorporated concrete stimulus dimensions by portraying the task as a problem of detection in which the participant was to decide which of several foods contained poison. A stimulus complex consisted of a meal with three different foods, and the feedback after the response indicated whether a person eating that meal had lived or died. After several "meals" involving various combinations of foods, the participant was asked to identify which food contained the poison.

The results with both abstract and concrete versions of concept-identification tasks have been quite consistent in indicating sizable age differences in the speed of acquiring the concept. Typical results are illustrated in Figure 5.2, with similar findings also reported by Arenberg (1968a), Hartley (1981), Nehrke (1973), and Wiersma and Klausmeier (1965). In all cases, it appears that older adults either require more trials to identify the concept, or are less accurate with a fixed number of trials, than young adults.

The reliability of age differences in concept-identification tasks seems indisputable in light of the consistent results from several independent studies. The interpretation of these findings is not quite so definitive, but it seems reasonable to conclude that older adults are less able to evaluate the relationships among different pieces of information and draw logical deductions than younger adults. A similar conclusion has been reached on the basis of results from a complex "logical analysis" task that requires the individual to determine the relationships between lights and buttons (e.g., Arenberg, 1974; Jerome, 1962; Young, 1966), and in a study of syllogistic reasoning (Nehrke, 1972). Friend and Zubek (1958) also reported sizable age-related declines for all five subtests of the Watson-Glaser Critical Thinking Appraisal Test which assess: (a) inference; (b) recognition of assumptions; (c) deduction; (d) interpretation; and (e) evaluation of arguments.

Ability to Discriminate Relevant from Irrelevant Information

In complex situations where there is a vast amount of information available but only a small portion that is pertinent to the issue at hand, the ability to distinguish between information that is, and is not, relevant is a very valuable characteristic. Many problems are overwhelming if one attempts to examine every little detail, but are relatively simple and straightforward when the

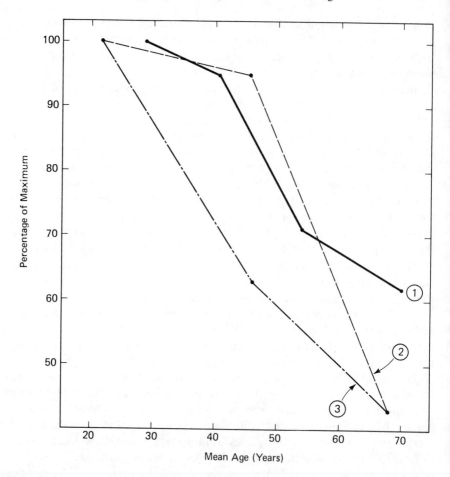

Figure 5.2. Concept identification performance at various ages expressed as a percentage of the maximum score across all ages. Numbers refer to different tasks or experiments: 1 = adapted from Brinley, Jovick, & McLaughlin (1974); 2 = adapted from Hayslip & Sterns (1979)—abstract problems; and 3 = adapted from Hayslip & Sterns (1979)—concrete problems.

critical variables have been isolated so that all other information can be ignored.

There have been frequent informal, almost anecdotal, reports in the literature on aging to the effect that older adults are less able to ignore irrelevant information than younger adults, but only a couple of research studies have directly addressed this issue. Rabbitt (1965a, 1965b) used a speeded classification task in which people had to make rapid decisions about the categorical identity of simple stimulus patterns. His major finding was that the age differences tended to increase as the number of stimulus dimensions irrelevant to the classification increased, suggesting that older adults had greater difficulty ignoring irrelevant information. (But see Chapter 8 for additional discussion of this result.)

A more recent study by Hoyer, Rebok, and Sved (1979) found essentially the same pattern of results as Rabbitt in a simple concept-identification task. Twenty young (mean age 21 years), 20 middle-aged (mean age 52 years), and 20 elderly (mean age 73 years) adults attempted to select which of two stimulus patterns was the most similar to a target stimulus pattern. The concepts were always defined in terms of one dimension (e.g., color, shape, number, or position), but zero, one, two, or three of the remaining dimensions could be variable and irrelevant. If an irrelevant dimension, i.e., a dimension other than the concept dimension, was not variable it still existed in the patterns but all stimuli had the same value on that dimension. For example, a problem with two irrelevant dimensions might consist of two gray squares in a vertical arrangement as the target, with four white squares in a vertical arrangement as one stimulus alternative, and three black triangles in a vertical arrangement as the other stimulus alternative. With this problem, shape would be the relevant dimension defining the concept, number and color would be the irrelevant variable dimensions, and positional arrangement would be the irrelevant constant dimension.

Individuals in all three age groups tended to commit more errors and take more time to make their decisions as the number of irrelevant dimensions increased. That is, the difficulty of determining which dimension was common to the target and one of the stimulus alternatives increased as the number of variable dimensions increased. Of greatest importance in the present context is that the differences among the age groups also became larger as the number of irrelevant dimensions increased from zero to three. In other words, the older adults seemed to have more problems in distinguishing between relevant and irrelevant dimensions than young and middle-aged adults. A slightly different experiment by Rebok (1981) failed to find an age difference in the effects of amount of irrelevant information, however, and thus this conclusion must be considered somewhat tentative.

Concrete and Abstract Thinking

One prerequisite of being able to profit from one's experience is the ability to think in the abstract rather than always in concrete terms. Only if one is able to discard the inessentials and retain the abstract principles will it be possible to transfer knowledge from an old familiar context to a new and different context. Abstraction can thus be considered the mechanism by which general, as opposed to specific, knowledge is acquired.

The status of the concrete-abstract distinction in aging research is much like that of the relevant versus irrelevant distinction discussed in the previous section; there is remarkable consensus on the basis of incidental and anecdotal evidence, but very few research studies have directly addressed this question. The prevailing opinion is that thinking becomes less abstract and more concrete with increased age.

Many authors have relied on unsystematic observations or researchers' speculations as the basis for their opinions, but there does seem to be at least one study providing rather direct evidence. This was a study by Bromley (1956) in which he asked adults of different ages to interpret proverbs. Bromley felt that this was an ideal procedure for assessing abstract thinking since the proverbs are expressed in concrete terms but they embody an abstract principle. If the individuals are able to think at an abstract level they will provide a general principle as their response. On the other hand, if they are limited to concrete thinking, very specific responses or even paraphrases of the proverb will be produced. Bromley employed both a free-response test, in which the participant provided the answers, and a multiple-choice test, where the participant selected the best answer from among three alternatives. The tendency to produce or select abstract and general responses decreased successively across age groups with mean ages of 27, 47, and 67 years. The very similar pattern with both types of tests is particularly interesting since it suggests that the age deficiency is not simply a difficulty in generating abstractions, but also in recognizing them among more concrete alternatives.

Ability to Proceed Systematically towards a Problem Solution

A final desirable characteristic for a decision maker is that he or she progresses in a systematic fashion to the eventual conclusion or solution, appropriately using information at every intervening stage. One who ignores relevant information, who fails to grasp the significance of information, or who alternates in an apparently haphazard fashion between various solution strategies, would obviously not command much respect as a decision maker.

Several researchers have reported that older adults seem less able than young adults to adopt and maintain an appropriate solution strategy. Young (1966), in particular, noted this tendency and attempted to train adults to employ an effective strategy. She found that the older adults were less consistent in their adherence to a strategy even when it was explicitly pointed out to them. Sanford (1973) in a search task, and Jerome (1962) and Arenberg (1974) in a logical-analysis task, also found reduced utilization of effective strategies among older adults.

Perhaps the clearest case of this age difference in solution strategy is evident in the results of an experiment by Offenbach (1974). A modified concept-identification task was used in which special stimuli without feedback were presented after every feedback trial. The purpose of the no-feedback presentations was to allow the participant's hypothesis about the concept identity to be determined without causing a change in that hypothesis. With 20 college students (mean age 19 years), Offenbach found that 88.4% of the hypotheses were retained after a correct trial, but only 9.4% were retained after an incorrect trial. In both respects these values are reasonable as one should keep a hypothesis that has been confirmed, but should discard a hypothesis that has been falsified. The older adults (mean age 75 years), however, were less consistent in following this strategy as they retained only 49.5% of hypotheses that had been confirmed, but 20.0% of the hypotheses that had been disconfirmed. Obviously the data indicate that the older adults in this study were less systematic in their progress towards the solution than the young adults.

Sanford (1973) reported a similar result in an analysis of strategies for locating a hidden target. The older adults (mean age 75 years) were much less likely than young adults (mean age 20 years) to employ a systematic stepwise search strategy, and more often relied on a haphazard, random, search pattern.

Sanford and Maule (1973) performed two experiments comparing the development of optimal prediction strategies in young (mean ages 20–22 years) and old (mean ages 64–70 years) adults. In both cases the older individuals used optimal strategies less often than did the younger ones. Maule and Sanford (1980) later confirmed this result in an experiment involving slightly different procedures.

The consistency of the finding that older adults are less systematic in their progress towards a problem solution suggests that this is a real phenomenon. If it were simply a chance result it is highly unlikely that the same trend would be evident across such varied tasks as logical analysis, concept identification, visual search and prediction. It therefore seems reasonable to conclude that with increased age there is a decline in the systematic nature of one's solution attempts.

Miscellaneous Factors

In addition to the attributes mentioned above, a number of other characteristics of older problem-solvers have been discussed as contributing to their poor performance in problem-solving and decision tasks. Friend and Zubek (1958), Welford (1958), and Young (1966), for example, have claimed that older adults are more likely than young adults to react to the content of propositional statements rather than the logical relationships in an argument. In Young's words, the behavior of the elderly is often dominated by "attitude rather than analysis." While these observations are interesting, it is not yet clear whether the emotional reactions are the cause, or simply a consequence, of the poor performance on logical tasks. The realization that a logical argument is quite complex may lead some individuals to ignore the abstract relationships and concentrate on the concrete content of the statements. However, at least one study (Nehrke, 1972) has reported that older adults are not differentially affected by the emotional content of a syllogism.

Another frequently mentioned characteristic of older problem solvers is that they experience more memory failures than younger people. This is manifested in a variety of ways, ranging from redundant inquiries in the 20-questions task (e.g., Denney & Palmer, 1981) and the button-light arrangement task (Arenberg, 1974; Jerome, 1962; Young, 1966), to great confusion with array sum tasks (e.g., Clay, 1956b). We will see in Chapters 6 and 7 that memory problems in older age are quite well documented and thus it is reasonable that an older adult will be impaired with problems and decisions that require reliance on memory.

Excessive cautiousness has also been frequently discussed as a factor contributing to poorer decision making in older adults. Two different procedures have been used to assess cautiousness, but one of them, the choice-dilemmas questionnaire, seems to measure reluctance to respond more than cautiousness per se (e.g., Botwinick, 1969; Okun, 1976), and thus it will not be discussed in this context.

The other procedure more directly assesses risk-taking propensities by instructing adults to attempt to solve problems (e.g., provide definitions of words) at the level of difficulty at which they feel comfortable. The measure of willingness to take risks is some index of the problem difficulty selected by the individual. The assumption is that an individual who selects a very high level of difficulty is more willing to take risks than an individual who prefers a lower level of difficulty. A problem with this assumption is that it is probably reasonable only if there is some special incentive to select the riskier alternative. For example, most natural high-risk situations also present much higher payoffs and thus selection of the riskier alternative leads to the possibility of a greater payoff. In two studies with a constant expected value (i.e., probability of success multiplied by the payoff for success) across difficulty levels (e.g., Okun & DiVesta, 1976; Okun & Siegler, 1976), it was found that adults in their 60s and 70s selected less difficult problems than adults in their late teens and 20s. However, when expected values varied across difficulty levels such that much higher rewards were given for greater levels of difficulty, no age differences were found in the difficulty level selected. (i.e., Okun & Elias, 1977). Taken together, these studies seem to indicate that when a special incentive is provided for selecting risky alternatives, as is the case with most real-life situations, little or no age differences are apparent.

Cognitive Regression

A very influential perspective in the child portion of the life span has been Piaget's Genetic Epistemology Theory of Cognitive Development in which the growth of knowledge in an individual was explained in terms of a series of qualitatively distinct cognitive structures or modes of logical organization. The existence of these cognitive structures, and the transition from one to another, was inferred from the responses of the child to a very cleverly designed set of tasks now familiar to all introductory psychology students (e.g., multiple classification, conservation, seriation, spatial egocentrism).

The structures (and hence competence on the tasks indexing these structures) were assumed to be acquired in a sequential fashion such that higher structures could only be obtained after the more primitive structures had been mastered. The Piagetian perspective has been extended to adult development by researchers postulating that increased age might be associated with a cognitive regression, i.e., a loss of cognitive structures during advanced age in the reverse order that they were acquired during childhood. Several early studies did indeed find some evidence for this hypothesis in that the tasks mastered latest in childhood were the first to exhibit declines in adulthood (see Hooper & Sheehan, 1977, and Papalia & Bielby, 1974, for reviews), although subsequent research with more comparable samples of individuals across the age span has generally failed to find significant age differences on Piagetian tasks (e.g., Chance, Overcast, & Dollinger, 1978; Muhs et al. 1979; Selzer & Denney, 1980; Tesch, Whitbourne, & Nehrke, 1978).

In addition to the weak empirical support for the regression phenomenon, at least two major problems with this hypothesis can be identified. One of these is that regression is not an intrinsic part of Piaget's developmental theory and substantial modifications would therefore be necessary to incorporate a reversal of the processes of accommodation and assimilation to produce a deterioration of cognitive structures. A more likely interpretation of the findings from a Piagetian perspective (e.g., Bearison, 1974) is that they simply reflect a growing discrepancy between the individuals' competence (which is still intact), and his or her performance (which is limited by a variety of structure-independent processes). This is clearly a less dramatic hypothesis than the view that the logical structures responsible for thought have regressed to an earlier primitive form, but it seems to be more parsimonious and consistent with the rest of Piaget's theory than the structural reversal hypothesis.

A second problem with the use of Piagetian tasks to infer a regression of qualitative thought modes is that the tasks used to index progressively more advanced cognitive structures are themselves systematically increasing in difficulty, and it is reasonable to expect that aging will affect difficult tasks earlier and to a greater extent than easy tasks. This trend would be consistent with a reversal of the normal developmental sequence, but it might simply be a reflection of the general tendency for age effects to be most pronounced on the most difficult activities. In other words, the finding that age differences are more apparent on difficult (i.e., developmentally later) tasks may have nothing to do with a change in cognitive structures.

If the Piagetian tasks are merely considered as a set of progressively graded cognitive tests, they should be evaluated with the same criteria applied to other tasks or tests in the literature. In this respect they do not fare very well. Compared to psychometric tests of the type discussed in Chapter 4 the Piagetian tasks are of unknown reliability and validity in adults. And compared to other laboratory-based measures of cognition such as those reviewed in this and subsequent chapters the Piagetian tasks are generally less analytical about the specific processes responsible for deficient performance. For all of these reasons, therefore, the Piagetian approach to adult cognition has not had a major impact in the field and hence it will not receive further discussion in this book.

The Critical Role of Experience

It is a fact that the majority of important decision-making positions in government and industry are held by adults in their 50s, 60s, and 70s. Since it is highly unlikely that these individuals would hold such responsible positions if they were not respected for their problem-solving or decision-making abilities, we are faced with something of a paradox. On the one hand, we find that it is primarily older adults who are in the highest-level decision-making positions, suggesting that some aspect of decision making tends to improve with age. On the other hand, the laboratory investigations summarized earlier in this chapter generally indicate that older adults perform worse, rather than better, than young adults on a variety of decision-making and problem-solving tasks. The key to this paradox seems to lie in the factor of experience. Increased age is associated with more and broader experience, and this greater experience apparently more than compensates for any other age-related limitations in most real-life decision contexts. All of the results discussed in this chapter must therefore be interpreted with considerable caution because at the present time there is no way to assess the relative contributions of experience versus "pure" ability in a given decision situation.

One example of the role of compensatory experience in problem solving comes from a recent analysis of chess players of varying ages by Charness (1981a, 1981b). Lehman (1953) and Elo (1965) have found that chess skill seems to peak in the decade of the 30s, with performance declining at greater ages. Charness was interested in determining whether different mechanisms might be employed to accomplish the same global performance (i.e., reach a comparable level of skill), and thus he selected a sample of 34 chess players ranging in age from 16 to 64 years, but with almost no correlation (i.e., $r = .09$) between age and chess skill.

Several chess-related tasks were administered to all participants and analyses performed to determine the influence of the age and skill level of the participant on task performance. Not surprisingly, because the sample was deliberately selected to have little correlation between age and skill, skill level but not age was a significant determinant of performance on tasks most clearly related to actual chess activity, e.g., selecting a move and predicting a game outcome. The more interesting results were that increased age was negatively related to ability to recall the locations of chess pieces in an unexpected recall task, and to the extensiveness of the mental search of plausible moves. (The latter measure was derived from an analysis of the taped records of participants attempting to select a move while thinking aloud.) The possibility that these measures are not relevant to actual chess performance was rejected by the finding that performance on both tasks was positively related to skill level. Similar results, although on a somewhat smaller scale, were also reported in an analysis of bridge players (Charness, 1979), and an independent sample of chess players (Charness, 1981c).

The implication of these results is that good performance in chess is usually associated with accurate recall of piece locations and extensive search of alternative moves, but that older players can achieve the same overall level of chess performance without high proficiency in these component skills. Although Charness (1981a) suggests that older players compensate by developing more efficient search processes, the evidence that this is the only, or the major, compensatory process employed by the older adults is not yet conclusive. What is quite clear, however, is that experience can lead to dramatic changes in the means by which a molar activity is performed, and thus age-related deficiencies in component activities may not be useful predictors of overall performance.

Theoretical Evaluation

Several investigators (e.g., Gardner & Monge, 1977; Wiersma & Klausmeier, 1965) have advocated a version of the disuse theory in attempting to account for age differences in certain problem-solving or decision-making skills. Gardner and Monge (1977) suggested that older people might be ". . . rusty at 'school-learned skills,' " and Wiersma and Klausmeier (1965) argued that the infrequency of new learning experiences might be reflected in "forgetting how to learn" in older individuals. While these types of explanations may apply to one or two limited abilities, they do not seem to have general applicability in the area of decision making. Laboratory tasks of decision making and problem solving are usually somewhat unfamiliar, but the abilities measured are presumed to be similar to those used in a great variety of daily activities. Indeed, Friend and Zubek (1958) found sizable age declines in a test of critical thinking specifically designed to involve practical and realistic problems. To the extent that the laboratory tests are valid reflections of daily decision-making and problem-solving activities, it seems unlikely that a disuse mechanism could explain the age differences that are typically observed.

At least two sources of evidence might be cited in favor of the disuse interpretation, but both have methodological flaws that limit their value. Denney and Palmer (1981) reported that the age decline started later and was more gradual for a task involving "practical problems" than for a traditional

(20-questions) problem-solving task. However, examination of the types of problems and scoring procedures in the practical-problems task suggests that personality or other factors may be more important than problem-solving ability in this task. As an example, one of the nine problems in the test was stated as follows:

> If you were walking down the street at night and saw two men beat up another man, take his wallet, and run, what would you do?

According to the scoring scheme described by the authors, more points were given for solutions that involved self-action than for those involving reliance on others. In the situation described above, therefore, one would apparently receive a lower score for calling the police than for attempting to intervene oneself, regardless of the size and strength of the assailants!

The practice of using more realistic tasks or materials than typically found in laboratory tasks thus runs the risk of introducing other contaminating factors that make interpretations difficult if not impossible. Moreover, without more information about the reliability and validity of such "practical" or "relevant" tasks it is simply impossible to arrive at any meaningful conclusions.

A second source of data sometimes mentioned as evidence for an experiential basis of age deficits in problem-solving ability comes from intervention studies attempting to modify problem-solving behavior of older adults. The logic of the argument seems to be based upon the idea that if it can be demonstrated that problem-solving performance of elderly adults can be improved by various manipulations such as strategy training, social reinforcement, practice, etc., then one can conclude that the age deficits typically observed are at least partially attributable to a lack of recent experience. However, most research of this type has employed only a single (elderly) age group, and as we have noted in previous chapters, without at least one other age group the results are of little or no value for explaining age differences. If it is to be argued that the intervention manipulation was responsible for age differences in the task, then it must be demonstrated that the intervention is helpful only (or at least to a significantly greater extent) for the older adults who are presumably deficient in that mechanism. If the younger individuals exhibit comparable performance improvements with the intervention then it cannot be claimed that the intervention mechanism is responsible for the initial differences between young and old adults.

A biological interpretation of the age differences also has difficulty because there is very little known about the neural processes responsible for such complex mental activity as decision making or problem solving. One possibility, mentioned by Rabbitt (1977) and Welford (1958), is that an age difference in some elementary neural process could, by a "vicious spiral effect," lead to progressively larger and more serious age differences in complicated activities that rely on that elementary process. For example, if the time for each mental operation is slowed with increased age, perhaps because more information samples are needed to compensate for the lower signal-to-noise ratio, older adults might experience: (a) greater difficulty in preserving relevant information while making decisions (because some information is lost while other information is being acquired); (b) fewer infrequent or "creative" solutions to problems (because each solution requires a greater proportion of the limited time for its generation); and (c) less organization of the problem information (because the greater time for information assimilation leaves less time for organization). This type of "domino effect" interpretation of age differences in complex mental activity is currently highly speculative, but it does provide an illustration of how a theory from the biological class of theories might be applied to this area.

The research by Charness on chess skill can be interpreted as evidence that performance in at least some situations accurately reflects competence since the chess players would be strongly motivated to make maximum use of their abilities in order to perform well in chess. Despite this incentive, age-related declines were observed in two relevant components of overall skill. Admittedly this is rather weak evidence, but there does not appear to be any other evidence either for or against the view that actual performance accurately reflects true competence at the present time.

It also appears premature to attempt to evaluate the general versus specific dimension for theories of problem solving and age because of the lack of sufficient data. A large-scale study employing a variety of problem-solving and decision-making tasks administered to the same individuals might prove useful in this regard as the intertask correlations would be informative about the feasibility of theories stressing a single, general mechanism.

To summarize, there is very little that can be said about the type of theory that might be successful in accounting for age-related differences in decision making and problem solving. Research that is more focused on theoretical issues is needed before one can determine whether a theory incorporating notions of disuse or concepts such as neural noise will be more successful in this area of research.

Summary

Many of the laboratory measures of problem-solving or decision-making skill can be criticized, but several broad conclusions nevertheless seem warranted. Older adults compared to young adults: are less likely to produce unusual solutions to problems; experience more difficulty in shifting from one type of problem to another; tend to form primitive "functional" organizations of items; have greater difficulty in ignoring irrelevant information; are less systematic in their progress towards a solution; require more information to make logical deductions; and may operate less effectively at abstract, as opposed to concrete, levels of thought. Whether we label these differences with terms such as creativity, flexibility, etc., is really immaterial to the fact that the differences do seem to exist and that they probably contribute to difficulties in decision making and problem solving. It is unfortunate that there has been little attempt to identify the specific processes responsible for age-related declines in reasoning since the measures obtained in psychometric intelligence batteries (e.g., see Figures 4.13 and 4.14) indicate that substantial age differences also exist in this type of decision making.

The role of experience in compensating for these age-related declines in basic skills was briefly discussed in the context of the recent research on chess players by Charness (1981a, 1981b, 1981c). There is still far too little information available about the positive contributions of experience, and thus it is quite possible that the results from inexperienced individuals have little generalizability to most actual decision situations where experience is typically positively correlated with age.

Because decision making and problem solving are so pervasive in our daily lives it seems unlikely that a disuse explanation could account for many of the age differences that have been observed in this field of research. However, it cannot yet be concluded that biological factors, e.g., in the form of an age-associated increase in neural noise, are primarily responsible since there has been very little work linking neural processes to complex mental activity.

6. Comprehension and Use of Information

It is conventional to make a distinction between learning and memory when reviewing research related to the understanding and retention of previously presented information. The two processes are obviously related, because both are necessary to infer the existence of either, and thus the basis for the learning-memory distinction is often arbitrary. For example, Craik suggests that:

> ... "learning" may be thought of as referring to the acquisition of general rules and knowledge about the world, while "memory" refers to the retention of specific events which occurred at a given time in a given place. (1977, p. 385)

As Craik acknowledges, his classification is very similar to the semantic-episodic distinction originally introduced by Tulving (1972). A roughly comparable division will be used here to organize coverage of the research literature in this general area. In this chapter, "Comprehension and Use of Information," we will examine research concerned with language comprehension, and a variety of topics loosely related to information use, i.e., structural characteristics of semantic memory, rate of activation of stored information, metamemory, and long-term or remote memory. In the following chapter, "Acquisition and Retention," more traditional memory research will be reviewed in which simple verbal material is tested for verbatim retention at relatively short intervals. The present chapter titles do not contain such familiar terms as "learning," "memory," "semantic," etc., but it is believed that they form a more meaningful basis for organization, and are more descriptive of the actual topics discussed, than most alternatives. There is also a pragmatic reason for not simply titling the present chapter "Learning" and the following chapter "Memory." Despite the obvious importance of learning processes throughout adulthood, there has been very little research on the long-term (i.e., greater than 1 day) acquisition of meaningful material as a function of adult age and consequently there is not yet much research that can be reported on learning processes, per se.

Comprehension

It was suggested in Chapter 4 that although most psychometric tests indicate that verbal ability is well maintained in later years, more demanding tests might reveal sizable age-related declines. Indeed, it was reported that older adults are generally poorer than young adults in tests of verbal fluency, classification, and verbal analogies. A verbal ability only briefly mentioned earlier but perhaps the most important in many daily activities is comprehension. Here it is not so much static world knowledge or information about the meaning of individual words that is critical, but rather the rapid integration of this intrinsic or old (stored) information with the extrinsic or new (message) information. Regardless of the vastness of one's store of information, comprehension is going to be impaired if one cannot activate that information at a rate commensurate with the pace of new external information.

The special status of comprehension among verbal abilities was demonstrated many years ago in an experiment reported by Thorndike et al. (1928). Young (mean age 22 years) and middle-aged (mean age 41 years) adults of comparable general intelligence received instruction in the Esperanto artificial language. Before and after the 20 hours of study four tests were administered assessing vocabulary, ability to follow written directions, ability to follow oral directions, and ability to understand written paragraphs, all involving the Esperanto language. At the initial testing the middle-aged and young adults performed equivalently on the vocabulary and written directions tests, with the middle-aged adults slightly inferior on the oral directions and paragraph tests. By the final testing both groups had improved substantially on all tests except following oral directions. In this test the young adults performed 109% better after the study period, but the middle-aged adults improved only 28%. Comparable improvement therefore occurred in the verbal tests that did not have time limits, but the increase was much less in middle-aged individuals with oral (externally paced) presentations requiring conversational response times (i.e., 5 sec). This finding suggested that the processes of simultaneous activation and integration of information involved in comprehension may present particular problems with increasing age.

Unfortunately, while this is clearly an important research area, there are presently only a limited number of studies that have investigated comprehension processes across the adult life span. The studies that do exist can be roughly classified into two categories, descriptive and analytical.

Descriptive Studies

Descriptive studies encompass all investigations that compared adults of varying ages on some measure of immediate understanding or comprehension of verbal material. Results from such studies have been fairly consistent, but not very informative. The consistency is that whether the material is spoken (e.g., Botwinick & Storandt, 1974a; Cerella, Paulshock, & Poon, 1982; Gilbert, 1941; Hulicka, 1966) or read (e.g., Gardner & Monge, 1977; Gordon, 1975; Gordon & Clark, 1974a; Moenster, 1972; Taub, 1976), and whether comprehension is assessed with procedures based on recall (e.g., Botwinick & Storandt, 1974a; Gilbert, 1941; Glanzer et al. 1958; Gordon & Clark, 1974a; Hulicka, 1966) or multiple-choice (e.g., Gordon, 1975; Gordon & Clark, 1974a; Moenster, 1972; Taub, 1976), older adults have been found to be less accurate in reporting information from immediately presented material. There are some exceptions to this trend (e.g., Feier & Gerstman, 1980), but by far the majority of the studies have indicated an age-related decline in the report of just-presented information.

To many readers the suggestion that increased age is associated with problems of comprehension may be surprising, and in apparent conflict with one's own observations of the reading and conversational abilities of older adults. This apparent contradiction is probably attributable to the large degree of redundancy in natural language. Redundancy, or duplication of information, exists at the lttr lvl, at __ word _____, and even at the level of sentences and entire phrases, _____ __ _____ __. The general meaning of the communication is usually evident without the necessity of registering and comprehending every word. Under controlled situations, however, hidden difficulties may become more obvious as the time of presentation is restricted or detailed information is requested in the test of comprehension.

As evident from the preceding survey, the descriptive studies have been reasonably consistent in reporting reduced comprehension performance with increased age. The low informativeness of these studies is a consequence of the absence of manipulations that would allow one to determine why older adults have this difficulty in comprehension.

Analytical Studies

The studies that can be classified as analytical have incorporated deliberate experimental manipulations to assess the nature of the comprehension deficit, but they appear at first glance to be somewhat inconsistent. The primary manipulation has been whether information probed in the comprehension test was explicit in the presented material, or was merely implied. Cohen (1979, 1981) reported that older adults relative to young adults had more difficulty with implicit than with explicit information, but Belmore (1981) reported exactly the opposite result.

Before attempting to resolve this discrepancy, we will first consider the experiments of Cohen, which at least are consistent with one another. Cohen's research strategy has been to administer a number of distinct tasks to the same young and old individuals, matched on vocabulary and digit span performance, and then to treat each task as a separate experiment. No details are provided in either the 1979 or 1981 reports concerning the order of task administration or the existence of possible fatigue effects, but this procedure does eliminate the worry that sample characteristics are fluctuating across experiments (or tasks).

The major conclusion reached by Cohen was that comprehension problems associated with increased age are a consequence of older adults being unable to access and integrate old stored information while simultaneously registering the surface meaning of newly presented information. In support of this thesis Cohen offered evidence from five experiments. One source of evidence (1979, Exp. 1) was that young (mean age 24 years) and old (mean age 68 years) adults did not differ in their accuracy of answering verbatim (explicit information) questions, but that older adults were much poorer at answering inference (implicit information) questions. A related finding (1981, Exp. 2) was that young (mean age 23 years) and old (mean age 69 years) adults were comparable at answering questions from text containing explicit information, but the elderly were greatly disadvantaged at answering questions from (implicit) text arranged such that the reader must infer the relevant information. Other results in support of the inadequate simultaneous processing interpretation were: (a) the finding (1979, Exp. 2) that older adults are less accurate than young adults at detecting anomalies between stored and presented information; (b) the discovery (1979, Exp. 3) that older adults apparently cannot identify the most important summary propositions as well as young adults because they do not retain as many gist facts from a story; and (c) the observation (1981, Exp. 1) that age differences are more pronounced with spoken than with written presentation, presumably because the latter allows more time for performing integration of old and new information than the former.

In contrast to Cohen, Belmore (1981) reported the results of only one experiment with a single sample of young (mean age 18 years) and old (mean age 67 years) adults. The participants in Belmore's study were required to read a three-sentence paragraph, and then decide whether a test sentence was true or false. The test sentence was designed to represent either paraphrase (explicit) information, or inference (implicit) information. Accuracy in an immediate test was quite high, ranging from 87% to 93%, and rather surprisingly, did not differ between inference and paraphrase questions. The older adults performed less accurately than the young adults with both types of questions, but the age difference was greater with paraphrase than with inference questions.

Most previous researchers employing samples of young adults, and Cohen (1979, 1981) with both young and old adults, have reported an advantage for explicit information relative to implicit information, and thus Belmore's failure to find such a result should make one cautious in interpreting her findings. It is not clear why Belmore was unable to replicate the basic phenomenon, but regardless of the reason it is difficult to evaluate arguments about age differences in the susceptibility to an effect when the effect is not evident in either age group.

Another reason for emphasizing the Cohen results rather than those of Belmore is that a series of experiments by Till and Walsh (1980) also indicate that older adults have difficulty with implicational information. Till and Walsh used a cued-recall task in which the cue presented at the time of recall was an implication of the sentence that was to be remembered. As an example, *The youngster watched the program* served as a to-be-remembered sentence with the implicational cue of *television.* To the extent that the individual has access to this implication of the sentence, the cue should facilitate recall of the sentence compared to when no cue was provided (free recall). This is exactly what happened across six conditions in three separate experiments for young (ages 17–31 years) adults. In contrast, the older (ages 57–81 years) adults actually had worse, rather than better, recall in the presence of the cue in all but one condition of one experiment. (That condition involved the participants writing a word reflecting their comprehension of the sentence at the time of its initial presentation.) The results of Till and Walsh (1980) are therefore inconsistent with Belmore's results, but quite consistent with the Cohen findings, i.e., with increased age there is a reduction in the spontaneous generation of implied information.

Three additional analytical comprehension experiments also give the impression of being in conflict. Meyer and Rice (1981) required adults in three age groups to read a 641-word passage and then: (a) write as much as they could remember from the passage; (b) complete an outline of the text; and (c) answer short questions about the material. Perhaps because both the reading and test phases were self-paced, no significant age differences were evident in the total number of idea units recalled or in the accuracy of either outline completion or question answering. However, a similar experiment by Zelinski, Gilewski, and Thompson (1980) with a shorter 227-word passage found significantly greater accuracy among young adults (ages 18–40 years) than older adults (ages 60–82 years). A difference in the range of information levels examined in the recall attempts may be contributing to this discrepancy as Meyer and Rice categorized recall idea units into 17 levels whereas Zelinski et al. (1980) apparently made only the 7 highest-level distinctions. Moreover, when Meyer and Rice examined the accuracy on levels 1 through 7 they did find a significant age advantage for the young adults, thus confirming the Zelinski et al. (1980) finding. Dixon, Simon, Nowak, and Hultsch (1982) also reported superior recall of important story items among young adults, and further demonstrated that the age differences persisted over a one-week interval. All three sets of results are therefore consistent with Cohen's findings that young adults are more accurate at recalling critical gist information, relative to supporting detail information, than are older adults.

Although there have not yet been many studies using analytical compre-hension or prose structure procedures, techniques such as these should be pursued further as they offer a promising tool for more precisely specifying the nature of the age deficit in meaningful comprehension processes.

Structural Characteristics of Semantic Memory

As noted earlier, Cohen has argued that older adults suffer comprehension problems because they are too slow in activating old information while simultaneously processing new information. An alternative possibility is that activation of stored information becomes ineffective, as well as merely inefficient, with increasing age. That is, older individuals may be unable to activate the old information, or to integrate old and new information, and not simply slower at handling these activities while also registering new information. This interpretation, that increased age is associated with a change in the structure or functioning of semantic memory, seems unlikely on the basis of at least four independent sources of evidence.

One class of evidence comes from the results of experiments by Walsh and Baldwin (1977) and Walsh, Baldwin, and Finkle (1980). Both experiments used a procedure introduced by Bransford and Franks (1971) to assess the abstraction and integration of linguistic ideas. This procedure involves the presentation and subsequent recognition of short sentences embodying from one to four basic ideas. During the acquisition phase of the experiment sentences that contain varying numbers of partial ideas are presented. In the test phase these and other sentences are presented with the instructions that the participant should judge whether each sentence had previously appeared in the acquisition phase. Many studies with young adults have reported that despite equal presentation frequencies, sentences embodying more partial ideas (e.g., three or four constituent ideas) are recognized better and with more confidence than sentences containing fewer partial ideas (e.g., one or two constituent ideas). Moreover, it is also generally found that this same trend is evident for both old (actually presented) and new (not previously presented) sentences. These findings have been interpreted as indicating that the original information was abstracted and integrated such that familiarity is no longer a function of actual presentation frequency, but instead is determined by the extent to which the test sentence matches the holistic, synthesized memory representation.

If the integration interpretation is accepted, one can consider the presence of a linear trend between recognition rate (i.e., accuracy and confidence) and number of partial ideas embodied in the test sentence as evidence of abstraction and integration. The major result in the Walsh and Baldwin (1977) and Walsh et al. (1980) experiments was that young (mean ages 19 years) and old (mean ages 67 and 74 years) adults exhibited comparable linear recognition trends. There were some differences across the two experiments, e.g., in the latter study the older adults were less accurate in answering comprehension questions in the acquisition phase and committed more false recognitions in the test phase, but the linear trend was evident in both age groups in both experiments. It therefore appears that older adults abstract and integrate linguistic information in a manner similar to young adults.

A second type of evidence indicating that there is not an age-related deficit in the functioning of semantic memory, in this case, activation of stored information, was provided by Howard, Lasaga, and McAndrews (1980). These investigators used a procedure adopted from Warren (1972) in which individuals attempt to name the color of ink in which a word is printed while simultaneously trying to remember words that are, or are not, related to the colored word. The reasoning is that holding words in memory may cause activation of related words which, in turn, may lead to temporary interference of color naming. Finding that related words in memory delays color naming more than unrelated words in memory would therefore constitute evidence that semantic activation occurred. The major result from the Howard et al. (1980) study was that three groups of adults (mean ages 31, 49, and 66 years) all exhibited this type of interference effect. The implication is that the process of activating stored information is effective at all ages.

A later experiment by these same investigators (Howard, McAndrews, & Lasaga, 1981) confirmed the basic finding with a different paradigm. The task in this second experiment involved making lexical decisions about whether two letter strings were both words. It has been reported with young adults that related words are classified more rapidly than unrelated words, and this has been attributed to a spreading activation, or priming, of related words in semantic memory. Howard et al. (1981) found that old (mean age 70 years) adults exhibited this effect in the same manner as young (mean age 28 years) adults, thus suggesting again that the activation process was unaffected by increased age.

Three studies employing a proactive-inhibition release procedure (see Wickens, 1972) have also demonstrated comparable activation of memorial information across age groups (Elias & Hirasuna, 1976; Mistler-Lachman, 1977; Puglisi, 1980). In her version of the procedure, Mistler-Lachman presented four successive triads of the same category of items (letters or digits in one experiment, boy's or girl's names in a second experiment), and then either presented another triad from the same category or from another category of items (e.g., digits if letters had previously been presented, or vice versa). The logic behind this procedure is that if performance differs between the two types of items on the fifth triad presentation then the participants must have been encoding the attribute of categorical membership of the stimulus. The normal accumulation of proactive inhibition associated with one category of items is apparently "released" when the stimulus material is shifted to a different category. Elias and Hirasuna (1976), Mistler-Lachman (1977), and Puglisi (1980) all found that both young and old adults exhibited proactive inhibition release, i.e., their performance differed between trials when the category remained the same and trials when the category was changed. The implication from this result is that young and old adults do not differ in the type of information encoded about a stimulus, but only in the amount of information.

Several miscellaneous experiments also support the idea that the activation of stored information only differs quantitatively, and not qualitatively, across age groups. The first of these experiments (Birren, 1955) examined verbal fluency by requesting adults of different ages to write as many words as possible from categories defined by the initial letter of the word. An analysis of relative word frequencies in the English language indicated that the greatest number of words began with the letter S, while the letter C was the first letter in only about 79% as many words, the letter N about 14%, and the letter Q approximately 5% as many words as the letter S. The rate of producing words across these categories can therefore be interpreted as a measure of the efficiency of accessing stored information of varying degrees of availability. However, because there is a well-documented age difference in speed of writing, the writing-speed variable has to be partialled out of later comparisons. This has been done in Figure 6.1 by expressing the values for each

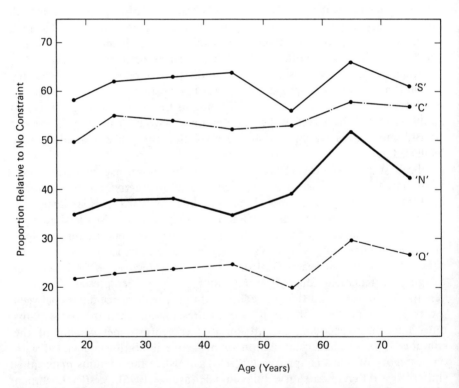

Figure 6.1. Number of words beginning with a specific letter written relative to the number of words beginning with any letter written at various ages. Data from Birren (1955).

category as a proportion of the total number of words written without restrictions on category membership, a measure of base writing speed. Between 28 and 127 individuals contributed to each data point.

The important finding from Figure 6.1 is that the relative efficiency of gaining access to both frequent and infrequent categories is approximately the same across all age groups. This suggests that the organization of stored information is similar across adulthood because, relative to their base writing speed, all age groups perform equivalently for accessible (e.g., S words) and inaccessible (e.g., Q words) categories in memory.

More recently, Mueller, Kausler, Faherty, and Oliveri (1980) compared classification speed of typical members of a category (e.g., ANIMAL-DOG) with atypical category members (e.g., ANIMAL-TADPOLE) in young (mean age 19 years) and old (mean age 71 years) adults. Older adults required 24% more time to make atypical than typical judgments, while two groups of younger adults required 27% and 37% more time. Because the older individuals were not impaired any more by the necessity of referring to rare members of a category, it can be inferred that the semantic storage system may be structurally similar in the two age groups. Bowles and Poon (1981), Eysenck (1975), Thomas, Fozard, and Waugh (1977) and Poon and Fozard (1980) also reported no interactions of age by exemplar typicality (Eysenck), or age by word frequency (Bowles & Poon, Poon & Fozard, Thomas et al.), again implying that adults of all ages were equally sensitive to the structural characteristics of semantic storage.

Considerably more research is necessary before one can be confident of conclusions about the reasons for age differences in comprehension, but the available evidence hints at an explanation. It appears that older adults have difficulty performing deep, integrative processes while simultaneously registering the surface meaning of either written or spoken messages. Moreover, the deficit seems not to be structural in nature since older adults have been found to be comparable to young adults in integration, activation, and access of information when that is the only task to be performed.

Rate of Information Activation

Most of the results discussed in the previous sections could be explained if it is assumed that with increased age there is a slower rate of accessing and utilizing memorial information. The derivation of implications would be hindered and comprehension impaired because of the greater time needed to retrieve relevant knowledge; but abstraction, integration, and activation of information would still be possible if time was not limited by presentation rate or rapid response requirements.

A number of procedures have been employed to measure the rate of activating stored information, but because of the age-related reduction in speed of most activities (cf. Salthouse, in press) it is rather difficult to obtain measures of activation rate independent of other factors. As an example, Thomas et al. (1977) and Poon and Fozard (1978) used a picture-naming procedure in which the time to name a picture is assumed to represent an estimate of the retrieval speed of verbal (name) information from long-term memory. The problem is that the naming task involves many components besides information retrieval, and longer naming latencies among older adults could be due to a slower retrieval component, or to a slowness in any of the other components.

These investigators did attempt to subtract out nonretrieval components by also using a matching task in which the picture was preceded by its name in order to eliminate the necessity of name retrieval. However, one can question the appropriateness of this procedure as a control for all nonretrieval components since there were a number of other differences between the matching and naming tasks (e.g., in matching there were two stimuli requiring attention instead of just one, and on half of the trials the experimenter "tricked" the participant by presenting a name that did not match the picture). Even more important than the appropriateness of the control task is the inconsistency obtained with this procedure. In the Thomas et al. (1977) study age differences were evident in both naming and matching tasks, with the former somewhat greater than the latter. Poon and Fozard (1978), on the other hand, reported that the age differences were not significant in the naming task, but were substantial in the matching task. There were a number of procedural differences across the two experiments that might be contributing to these discrepancies (e.g., the participants were somewhat older and the stimulus materials were more familiar in the Thomas et al. study), but whatever the reasons the present inconsistency of the findings necessarily leads to reservations about the usefulness of this particular technique.

A much better accepted and more frequently employed procedure for measuring the rate of accessing memorial information was developed by Sternberg (1969, 1975). His technique involves the presentation of a list of items (e.g., digits or letters) to be remembered, followed soon after by a probe stimulus that is to be rapidly classified with respect to whether it was in the earlier memory set. The results of literally dozens of experiments have revealed that reaction time to the probe stimulus increases in a linear fashion with increases in the number of items in the memory set. According to the model proposed by Sternberg (1969, 1975), the intercept of the memory set-reaction time function reflects the duration of processes of stimulus encoding, decision, and response preparation or execution, while the slope represents the time to scan (retrieve or activate) a memory representation.

For the present purposes the slope parameter is of greatest interest because it can be interpreted as an estimate of the time required to activate information in memory, independent of the duration of all other processes. At least seven experiments have been reported in which adults of different ages have been compared in the Sternberg paradigm, and all but one have reported an age-related increase in the slope of the memory set-reaction time function. The

single exception (Marsh, 1975) was primarily due to one atypical data point
in the data of older adults, apparently caused by incomplete understanding of
the task among some participants. The results of the remaining studies,
expressed in terms of the proportion of the fastest slopes, are illustrated in
Figure 6.2.

The important point to be noted from Figure 6.2 is that the time needed
to activate information from memory increases by over 60% between the ages
of 20 and 50. Extensive practice with the same stimulus items may reduce or
eliminate this age difference (e.g., Plude & Hoyer, 1981; Salthouse & Somberg,
1982c), but for up to moderate levels of experience (e.g., 200–2000 trials) there
appears to be a slower rate of accessing and utilizing stored information
among older adults.

There are undoubtedly other factors involved in the comprehension deficit

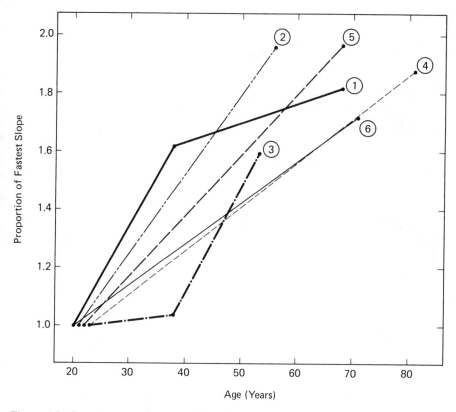

Figure 6.2. Sternberg memory-scanning slope at various ages as a proportion of the
fastest slope across all ages. Numbers refer to different experiments: 1 = adapted from
Anders, Fozard, & Lillyquist (1972); 2 = adapted from Anders & Fozard (1973); 3 =
adapted from Eriksen, Hamlin, & Daye (1973); 4 = adapted from Ford, Roth, Mohs,
Hopkins, & Kopell (1979); 5 = adapted from Madden & Nebes (1980); and 6 = adapted
from Salthouse & Somberg (1982a).

observed in older adults relative to young adults, but the slower rate of activating old information almost certainly plays a major role. If comprehending a message requires activation of memorial information and the duration of that activation process is longer with increased age, it is only to be expected that older adults will experience difficulties understanding spoken, or complex written, communications. Despite the plausibility of this interpretation, it must be admitted that at the present time it is primarily speculative and based on circumstantial rather than direct evidence. More research is needed to investigate possible age differences in the rate of performing actual comprehension processes such as encoding the meaning of a phrase, identifying possible implications, and evaluating potential inconsistencies with earlier presented information. Until such research is available it is impossible to reject the possibility that the existence of well-documented age differences in both comprehension and rate of information activation is mere coincidence, rather than a reflection of a true causal interconnection.

Metamemory

In many ways human memory can be considered analogous to a large information storage system like a library, and consequently it can be considered to be confronted with problems similar to those facing a librarian, e.g., supervising the organization of information, monitoring what is stored, and determining the most efficient methods of gaining access to information. Within the field of memory these executive functions have come to be called metamemory processes since they do not deal with specific information within memory, but rather with the operation of the memory system in general.

A question that has attracted considerable interest in recent years concerns the existence of possible age differences in metamemory, regardless of whether or not there are age differences in what already exists, or what can be deposited, in the memory store. The question has important implications for overall cognitive functioning since inefficient metamemory processes might exaggerate any memory differences that exist, while highly adaptive processes could conceivably compensate for deficits in other aspects of memory.

Much of the speculation about possible age differences in metamemory was fueled by reports that older adults use memory strategies less often, or less effectively, than young adults. Perhaps the most dramatic demonstration of this strategy difference is evident in a recent study by Sanders, Murphy, Schmitt, and Walsh (1980). These investigators were able to analyze strategies of rehearsal by instructing participants to "verbalize aloud everything they thought of as they studied." They found that young adults (mean age 24 years) rehearsed initial items from a list of related words in a serial fashion, and later list items in a categorical fashion. Both types of rehearsal are strategic, i.e., nonrandom, and can be considered optimal for that segment of the list. In marked contrast, the older adults (mean age 74 years) in this study exhibited no evidence of either type of strategy, and instead seemed to rehearse by simply naming each item as it was presented. These data are therefore quite clear in indicating that increased age is associated with a reduction in the use of memory strategies that might facilitate memory performance. Further research confirming this general finding will be discussed in Chapter 7; for the present it is sufficient to note that many other experiments have reported similar results.

The issue in metamemory is whether these age differences in strategy utilization, as just one example, are attributable to a lack of awareness about the existence or usefulness of the strategies, or to a fundamental inability to employ the strategies.

Among the procedures for investigating knowledge about memory processes, perhaps the most direct is simply to ask people about the kinds of memory difficulties they experience, and the strategies they employ, in their attempts to remember information. Perlmutter (1978) administered such a questionnaire to 32 adults between 20 and 25 years of age and to 32 adults between 60 and 65 years of age. She found no age differences either in general knowledge about memory, or in reported use of various mnemonic strategies.

Comparable performance across age groups has also been reported in a variety of laboratory tasks assessing metamemory functioning. For example, both Perlmutter (1978) and Murphy, Sanders, Gabriesheski, and Schmitt (1981), but not Bruce, Coyne, and Botwinick (1982), reported that young and old adults were equally accurate at predicting their level of recall in a subsequent task. The implication is that information about the state of one's own memory is equally available throughout adulthood. It is also noteworthy that young adults outperformed older adults in the recall tasks in all three experiments, and thus prediction accuracy may be maintained despite an overall reduction in memory performance.

Lachman, Lachman, and Thronesberry (1979) also reported age invariance in measures related to monitoring memory information. These researchers found that adults with mean ages of 21, 50, and 69 years all exhibited comparable trends with latencies, confidence ratings, and "feelings of knowing" for information not immediately recalled but later recognized in a multiple-choice test. That is, for all age groups these indicators revealed that the individual can differentiate between information not presently available for recall but stored in memory, and information unavailable for recall and not existing in memory. This outcome suggests that all age groups were aware of the relative accessibility of information in their memory stores, and that whatever other age-related memory problems that may exist are unlikely to be attributable to defective monitoring of stored information.

There is one recent finding that runs counter to this trend of finding no age differences in measures of metamemorial functioning. Murphy et al. (1981) examined a measure of the time spent studying material before attempting to recall and found that young adults (mean age 20 years) spent more time studying than older adults (mean age 69 years). Moreover, it was also reported that older adults performed in a manner similar to young adults if forced to spend as much time preparing for recall as the young adults. Still another finding was that the young adults exhibited greater variation in study time with shifts in task demand than did older adults. Murphy et al. (1981) interpreted these results as suggesting that there is an age decline in the monitoring of recall readiness, and in the flexibility with which one can modify the state of readiness.

There are at least three criticisms that can be directed at this work and the conclusion based upon it. The first is that four other studies have reported conflicting results. Bruce et al. (1982) and Perlmutter (1978, 1979a) found no age differences in study time, and Perlmutter, Metzger, Nezworski, and Miller (1981) found that older adults (mean age 64 years) actually took more time in preparation for subsequent recall than did young adults (mean age 20 years). The second criticism is that the greater variation in study time across tasks was obtained only with absolute measures of performance and was not evident in the arguably more meaningful proportional or relative measures. Finally, there is a curious anomaly in the results of the recall readiness phase as all individuals received list lengths based on their own memory spans, and yet the young adults were 11% more accurate than the older adults. The fact that the older adults decreased their performance so dramatically between the first and second testing of memory span while the young adults maintained roughly comparable performance suggests that other factors such as differential fatigue may have been operating in this study. For all of these reasons, therefore, it seems best to disregard the Murphy et al. (1981) results as they apply to metamemory functioning. The basic finding is apparently not reliable, and other aspects of the study make one hesitant about accepting any strong conclusions from these data.

Nickerson (1980) has pointed out two other aspects of memory functioning that should fall within the realm of metamemory, but which apparently have not yet received much investigation in adults of any age (however for a notable exception see Johnson and Raye, 1981). The first of these concerns the ability to distinguish between information (either current in the form of stimulation, or past in the form of memory) originating in the outside world, and that originating from within the organism. Loss of this ability results in profound psychological disturbances often requiring institutionalization, but virtually nothing is presently known about intermediate levels of this ability and whether or not it is affected by aging.

The second metamemorial process mentioned by Nickerson concerns what might be called prospective memory, the mental notes we make to ourselves in order to perform some activity in the future. How is it that we are able to remember to call Mr. Jones on Tuesday, or to bring milk home for dinner after being told in the morning before going to work? The fact that we sometimes fail to remember to perform such actions indicates that prospective memory of this type is fallible, but we do not yet know whether the degree of fallibility is related to adult age in any systematic fashion. Because this is likely to be one of the more salient aspects of memory in everyday life it would be desirable to investigate individual and developmental differences in prospective memory ability.

Research investigating the effects of adult age on metamemory processes is still very new and consequently only a very limited number of studies are currently available. As we have seen, most of the results from these studies suggest that there are not pronounced age differences in the monitoring processes investigated thus far. The existence of age differences in the frequency or effectiveness of strategy use still presents a challenge to the metamemory perspective since there have not yet been any direct explorations of whether older adults are as capable of selecting and utilizing these strategies as young adults. Stated differently, there is presently no basis for distinguishing between a performance-based explanation, as might be expected if a meta-memory process declined with age, and a competence-based explanation, in which case it is simply beyond the ability of the older adult to employ a strategy while also trying to remember.

Remote Memory

The use of stored information obviously involves a variety of memory processes. Memory is a topic that has had a long and active research history in psychology, and as a consequence a number of integrative theories or models have been developed in this area, several of which will be discussed in Chapter 7. However, an aspect of memory that has typically not been represented in theoretical conceptualizations but which is the subject of considerable folklore concerns memory about very remote (on the order of years or decades rather than minutes or hours) experiences. There are often reports of older individuals with phenomenal memories about events that occurred 40–60 years ago, but very poor memories for events of the last few minutes. This raises the question of whether memory problems associated with aging are confined to recent events, with the possibility that information about early experiences are immune from the effects of aging. Unfortunately, despite several attempts at investigating very long-term or remote memory, there is not yet enough evidence to allow an adequate evaluation of this hypothesis.

One source of "evidence" that can be easily dismissed are the anecdotal reports of the remarkable memories of older adults in recalling very old happenings. At least four problems limit the value of such reminiscences for scientific purposes. First, the information that is recalled is often impossible to verify and thus the memories may be more fiction than fact. Second, the individual in such situations is usually very selective in the report of infor-mation, and may simply be sampling only a few extremely salient pieces of information. Third, much of the information could be inference rather than memory. Schonfield and Stones (1979) illustrated this point with the example of an individual describing his or her fifth birthday by "remembering" that there were five candles on the cake. Obviously, certain facts would be extremely likely in particular contexts and their accurate description can often be inferred and need not be based on remembered information. The fourth problem with anecdotal reports as evidence for impressive long-term memory is that the information is likely to have been repeated many times, and thus the "memory" is only as old as the last repetition. If reminiscing is a favorite activity in family gatherings, the individual need only remember the information from one gathering to the next and not since the time of the original event.

Several investigators have devised questionnaires in an attempt to introduce more control into the assessment of very long-term memory. Generally the questions concern public events that occurred at different points in an individual's life span. This technique has the advantage of testing objectively verifiable events, and allowing the investigator to control the sampling of information at different periods. Important disadvantages of this approach are that it is not easy to ensure that items from different years were originally learned to the same degree, and that it is often impossible to be certain that no other opportunity for acquisition or rehearsal occurred since the original event. These problems can be illustrated by considering the following two questions from a fictitious remote memory questionnaire.

1. What happened on December 7, 1941?
2. Which baseball team won the World Series in 1955?

If items such as these were to appear on a remote memory questionnaire most individuals would probably be judged to have accurate memories of 1941, but rather poor memories for 1955. However, the fact that the event used to represent 1941 was much more important and salient to most people than the event used to represent 1955 would tend to invalidate this result. Most remote memory questions do not involve questions differing in importance or significance to the extent illustrated here, but the problem of unequal item difficulty or initial acquisition level across time periods is nevertheless a serious limitation of nearly all existing questionnaires.

The second problem, concerning the opportunities for later acquisition or rehearsal of information, is also illustrated by the preceding example. It is likely that many adults born after 1941 would correctly answer the first question, and yet the information could not possibly have been acquired from personal experience of the actual event. Other opportunities for acquiring that information must have been present or else the correct answer could not have been given. This indicates that items are probably inappropriate for a test of remote memory if people who were not even alive at the time of the critical event are able to score above a chance level. Unfortunately, most of the questionnaires that have been used in aging investigations fail to meet this criterion of chance performance by individuals too young to have acquired the relevant information by first-hand experience.

In view of these methodological problems, it is perhaps not surprising that the results from questionnaire studies of remote memory have been mixed. Two early reports indicated poorer performance among the older individuals in samples of age 40–90 (Warrington & Sanders, 1971) or age 50–90 (Squire, 1974). Botwinick and Storandt (1974a) reported no significant age difference across the age range 20–80, while Storandt, Grant, and Gordon (1978) and Botwinick and Storandt (1980) reported very complicated patterns with no easily interpretable age trend. Perlmutter (1978), employing the same questionnaire as Botwinick and Storandt (1974a), and Poon, Fozard, Paulshock, and Thomas (1979) with a different questionnaire, found older adults superior to young adults in memory for remote events.

No age differences were reported in a slightly different procedure in which examinees were asked for the dates and judgments of priority about events occurring 3–18, 43–58, or 103–118 years ago (Perlmutter, Metzger, Miller, & Nezworski, 1980). Because it was clearly impossible for the participants to have acquired all of the information through first-hand experience, this is better considered as a test of stored information than of memory. Performance was also very low, ranging from 1% to 7% correct on dates and 50% to 69% (where 50% is chance) on the priority judgments. In light of these factors, the results of the Perlmutter et al. (1980) study cannot be considered very informative about age differences in remote memory.

Still another technique has been reported by Franklin and Holding (1977) and McCormack (1979). These investigators used a free-association procedure in which the research participants were presented with single words and the instructions to provide an immediate association with a personal reference. The associations were then time-tagged with respect to the date of the event in one's life. Because there is no means of checking either the accuracy of the memory or the initial date of the relevant event, this technique seems to be of limited usefulness for studying remote memory. It has also provided rather conflicting results thus far in that Franklin and Holding (1977) found that the majority of associations produced by adults in their 70s were triggered by events in the last 20% of their life span, whereas McCormack (1979) reported the greatest frequency of associations dated from the first 25% of one's life.

The diversity of these results, in conjunction with the methodological difficulties hampering interpretation even with consistent results, makes it impossible to draw any conclusions from the research employing the questionnaire and related techniques. Two other techniques have recently been introduced, and although they too have problems, with modification they may eventually prove to be useful in aging research.

One of these alternative techniques was employed by Bahrick and his colleagues in two separate studies (Bahrick, 1979; Bahrick, Bahrick, & Wittlinger, 1975). In one study he assessed memory for names and faces of high school classmates, and in the other, memory for college campus locations. As one might expect, Bahrick found sizable performance declines as a function of interval since the experience (high school or college) with most types of information. Unfortunately, since nearly everybody has these experiences at approximately the same age, it is impossible with this procedure to separate losses due to the age of the memory (time since the experience), and those due to the age of the individual (chronological age at testing). This will obviously limit the applicability of such a technique for aging research. The confounding of age of memory and age of the individual is also a problem with a variant of this procedure in which individuals of different ages are asked to recall the names of former school teachers (e.g., Schonfield, 1972).

Another technique, which apparently has not yet been used in aging studies, is based on questions about television programs that appeared for only one season. Squire and Fox (1980) have recently summarized the evidence concerning the validity of this technique for assessing remote memory, but it will clearly be useful only for individuals who have been moderate to intense watchers of television, and can only be used for periods and cultural contexts in which television was widely available. A modification of this technique involving tests of memory for songs popular in different decades was administered to middle-aged (mean age 46) and older (mean age 65) adults by Bartlett and Snelus (1980). The older individuals were poorer at both melody and title recognition than the middle-aged individuals, despite the fact that some of the songs were popular before the middle-aged participants were even born.

An interesting experiment employing similar reasoning was reported by Speakman (1954), who contrasted adults of varying ages in their memory for discontinued stamp colors. After a period of nearly 20 months, memory for old stamp colors declined monotonically with increased age between 20 and 86 years. Although Speakman's results seem to indicate poorer remote memory with increased age, the findings should merely be considered suggestive because of the relatively small sample of participants and the absence of control over initial level of learning or familiarity with the stamp colors.

Despite the interest in remote memory and aging, we are not yet in a position to offer any conclusions. The procedures that have been employed are flawed, and have yielded very inconsistent results. Moreover, at the present time there do not appear to be any completely satisfactory procedures for assessing very long-term memory and thus this may be a topic which cannot be adequately investigated in the immediate future.

Theoretical Evaluation

Although there have been few investigations of adult age differences in learning across two or more sessions, it is from this type of research that most arguments about the viability of a disuse hypothesis are based. For example, one study often cited as support for a disuse interpretation of age differences in comprehension and utilization of information is the Sorenson (1930) comparison of adults of different ages taking the same college courses. Sorenson reported that performance in a course was independent of the student's age for adults who had recently taken other college courses, but increased age was negatively related to course performance for individuals returning to college after a long absence. The apparent conclusion is that learning skills may become "rusty" with disuse, but given an opportunity to sharpen or brush-up on those skills there is no effect of increased age on ability to learn.

However, a closer examination of some of the methodological details of this experiment serves to weaken one's confidence in the conclusion. One problem is that the classification of individuals as having had recent college courses or not was based entirely on the specific course the individuals were taking. One course was considered to consist primarily of school teachers returning to college after a long absence, while two other courses were assumed to contain individuals with recent college attendance. This classification is obviously very gross, and the fact that the age range was from 20 to 56 in the "long absence" group suggests that it was imprecise since it is highly unlikely that someone aged 20 could have had a "long absence" from formal schooling. The distribution of ages is another problem in that only 3% of the total sample was over 50 years of age, and 77% were 36 years of age or younger. This limited range obviously restricts the generalizations one can make to the entire adult life span. And finally, although the correlation between age and course performance was different from zero ($r = -.32$) in the "long absence" group, this correlation was not significantly different from that obtained in one of the courses containing "recent learners" ($r = -.12$). Taken together, these characteristics suggest that the Sorenson (1930) study is not very convincing evidence for the disuse interpretation.

The results of another set of early experiments can be interpreted as support for a biologically based deterioration of learning abilities, and indirectly as evidence against a disuse perspective. These were experiments by Thorndike et al. (1928) on what they termed "sheer modifiability." In order to study learning independent of previous experience, Thorndike et al. selected very simple activities such as drawing lines of specified lengths and writing with the wrong (nonpreferred) hand. The question of primary interest was how much improvement could be obtained with practice in groups of young (early 20s) and middle-aged (early 40s) adults. It was presumed that the degree of improvement could serve as an index of the "sheer modifiability" of the nervous system at different ages. By this criterion, basic learning ability was found to be impaired with increased age. The middle-aged adults reduced their line length errors by only 35% compared to the 53% error reduction in young adults, and they improved their rate of wrong-hand writing from 35% to 50% the rate of preferred-hand writing while young adults improved from 31% of their "normal" rate to 58% of that rate with comparable amounts of practice. The apparent implication is that the nervous system of older adults is not as malleable, and as amenable to new learning, as that of younger adults. The age differences were not particularly large, however, and since line drawing and wrong-hand writing are rather unusual activities one might have reservations about basing conclusions concerning learning ability on the results from such tasks.

With the exception of these very early studies, there is little basis for distinguishing between maturational and environmental interpretations of the age differences in the comprehension and use of information. There is no convincing evidence that environmental factors can account for the observed results, but there is also not yet any understanding of the neurological processes involved in these activities nor how they are affected by increased age.

Because of the nature of the processes examined in this chapter, it seems rather unlikely that the age differences that have been observed could be easily explained by assuming only a deficit in performance, and not competence, with increased age. For example, comprehension is a process involved in nearly all human interaction and it is implausible that one would perform at less than the maximum level of competence in such an important activity. Moreover, the evidence suggests that many of the age differences are more quantitative than qualitative, and thus it does not appear that the older adults are simply doing different things than young adults. The topic of metamemory was initially approached with the expectation that older adults would be found to be deficient in their knowledge about memory functioning and monitoring, but so far this expectation has not been confirmed. Because there are apparently not any pronounced age differences in the awareness of one's own memory operations it is unlikely, although certainly not impossible, that age differences in other aspects of memory performance are caused by unfamiliarity with mnemonic techniques rather than diminished competence.

The general-specific dimension is difficult to evaluate because of the wide range of topics discussed and the variable pattern of age trends. With respect to comprehension processes a single general mechanism, slower rate of information activation and integration, may account for nearly all of the reported findings. There are evidently no structural differences in the semantic memory systems of young and old adults, and it has been demonstrated that older adults require more time for memory activation than young adults. The situation concerning age differences in metamemory and remote memory is still unclear, and it remains to be seen whether a processing-rate mechanism would be able to account for any age differences that might be found in these processes.

Summary

The topics discussed in this chapter do not form a coherent whole, but instead consist of a variety of issues broadly related to the understanding and utilization, i.e., learning, of information. Comprehension processes were found to be impaired in older adults, apparently because of a growing inability to simultaneously register message information while also activating the meaning and implications of the information from a semantic storage system. Because older adults are sensitive to integration, associative-interference, proactive-inhibition-release, item-typicality, and item-frequency effects in the same manner as young adults, it seems unlikely that the comprehension difficulty is based on a structural disruption of the semantic storage system. Moreover, independent evidence confirms that the rate of activating information in memory decreases with increased age.

The means by which one organizes and controls memory processes was discussed under the topic of metamemory. Not much research is yet available concerning adult age trends in this area, but what does exist reveals little or no age differences. Older adults do seem to employ useful mnemonic strategies less frequently than young adults, but they apparently have equal awareness of the strategies, and are as accurate as young adults in assessing their level of confidence or predicting their degree of recall. Other interesting aspects of metamemory have not yet been investigated, and at the present time it is not known why certain mnemonic strategies are used less often or less effectively with increased age.

The final topic discussed was long-term or remote memory. Despite a number of recent studies, it was concluded that methodological problems inherent in all current techniques for assessing memory for long-term information make it impossible to reach any conclusions about the influence of age on memory for "old" information.

7. Acquisition and Retention

Although it is often referred to as if it were a single process, memory is not a unitary ability but instead consists of many diverse aspects with a variety of different age trends. One particularly dramatic illustration of how age selectively affects some facets of memory more than others is available in a contrast of the age functions for a paired-associate task and a digit-span task.

Paired-associate tasks require learning to associate stimulus-response pairs such that the individual will be able to produce the response term when the stimulus term is presented alone. Several different measures can be used to express paired-associate performance (e.g., number of trials to a given criterion, number of errors to criterion, and number of correct responses after a fixed number of trials), but for the current purposes all measures for a given age group have been expressed as a percentage (or its reciprocal in the case of errors or number of trials) of the maximum score across all age groups. Data from six different studies, each including at least 20 individuals in three or more age groups, are illustrated in Figure 7.1.

The digit-span task measures the maximum number of unrelated digits that can be immediately repeated in the original sequence. Performance on this task, expressed as a percentage of the maximum score across age groups, is illustrated in Figure 7.2. (The data of Figure 7.2 differ from those of Figure 4.7 in representing only forward digit span, whereas Figure 4.7 indicates the sum of forward and backward digit spans.)

The important point in comparing the age trends in Figures 7.1 and 7.2 is that they are quite different. Paired-associate performance appears to decline by as much as 20% to 40% between 20 and 70 years of age, while the difference on the digit-span task is slight to nonexistent. This type of divergence of age

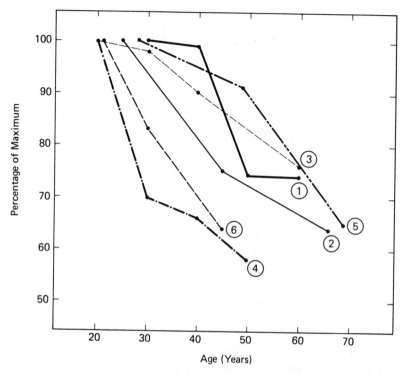

Figure 7.1. Paired-associate score at various ages expressed as a percentage of the maximum score across all ages. Numbers refer to different experiments: 1 = adapted from Canestrari (1968); 2 = adapted from Gladis & Braun (1958); 3 = adapted from Hulicka (1966); 4 = adapted from Monge (1971); 5 = adapted from Smith (1975); and 6 = adapted from Thorndike, Bregman, Tilton, & Woodyard (1928).

trends suggests not only that there are different kinds of memory, but also that some are more affected by increased age than are others.

Although the discrepancy between the age functions for the paired-associate and digit-span tasks serves to illustrate the point that different aspects of memory may be differentially influenced by aging, one should be very cautious in making across-task comparisons of this type. The problem is that it is generally impossible to equate the level of difficulty across tasks with different types of information and response requirements. For example, while the age trends in Figures 7.1 and 7.2 may be representative of most situations, it is a simple matter to construct a very easy paired-associate task that exhibits no age difference, and it might also be possible to increase the difficulty of the digit-span task such that it results in sizable differences with increased age. The problem of variations in task difficulty is particularly severe in making age comparisons because there is considerable evidence in support of the view that the magnitude of age differences varies directly with the level of difficulty of the task. That is, as task difficulty increases by increasing the memory

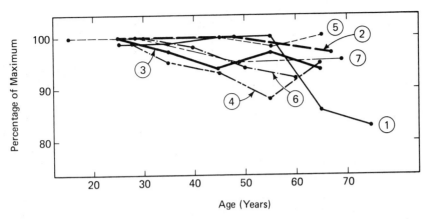

Figure 7.2. Digit span score at various ages expressed as a percentage of the maximum score across all ages. Numbers refer to different experiments: 1 = adapted from Botwinick & Storandt (1974a); 2 = adapted from Bromley (1958); 3 = adapted from Caird (1966); 4 = adapted from Inglis & Ankus (1965); 5 = adapted from Inglis & Caird (1963); 6 = adapted from Kriauciunas (1968); and 7 = adapted from Smith (1975).

demands, decreasing the familiarity of the material, requiring other concurrent activity, etc., performance generally declines more rapidly in older adults than in young adults.

This argument indicates that comparisons of the magnitude of age declines across various tasks (e.g., as reported in Botwinick & Storandt, 1974a; Gilbert, 1941; Gilbert & Levee, 1973) may be interesting, but not necessarily informative about the nature of the memory problems associated with increasing age. In order to obtain this latter information one must turn to research based upon modern analytical models of memory.

Before examining the research findings derived from recent memory models, we will consider a criticism often directed at contemporary research on memory. Skeptics frequently claim that the majority of research on memory is exclusively concerned with meaningless verbal material such as digits, nonsense syllables, or isolated words, and therefore it has little or no generalizability to the more realistic types of material found in natural learning environments. There are two rebuttals to this type of criticism—one methodological and one pragmatic. The methodological argument is that only by controlling the relevant material in this fashion can one be certain that the processes being investigated are related to current memory and not previous learning or experience. Most comparisons derived from naturalistic environments are of limited value because the achievement of high performance might be attributable either to prior familiarity with the material, or to superior learning and memory ability. Unless there is some degree of control over these factors any results one might obtain would be difficult to interpret because of the confounding of variables.

The pragmatic argument is that many studies have now demonstrated that age trends very similar to those found with meaningless verbal material are evident with other types of material. For example, sizable age-associated declines in the verbal recall, reproduction, or recognition of pictures, spatial displays, and geometrical drawings have been reported by Adamowicz (1976, 1978); Adamowicz and Hudson (1978); Arenberg (1977, 1978, 1982); Botwinick and Storandt (1974a); Bromley (1958); Ceci and Tabor (1981); Charness (1981b); Davies (1967); Farrimond (1967); Ferris, Crook, Clark, McCarthy, and Rae (1980); Gilbert and Levee (1971); Harwood and Naylor (1969); Heron and Chown (1967); Howell (1972); Kendall (1962); Laurence (1966); Mergler, Dusek, and Hoyer (1977); Murphy et al. (1981); Perlmutter, Metzger, Nezworski, and Miller (1981); Riege and Inman (1981); Riege, Kelly, and Klane (1981); Schear and Nebes (1980); Smith and Winograd (1978); Trembly and O'Connor (1966); Winograd and Simon (1980); and Winograd, Smith, and Simon (1982). Substantial age-related reductions in recognition or non-verbatim recall of meaningful verbal prose such as sentences, paragraphs, and recipes have been reported by: Botwinick and Storandt (1974a); Cohen (1979); Dixon et al. (1982); Gilbert (1941); Gilbert and Levee (1971); Gordon (1975); Gordon and Clark (1974a); Hulicka (1966); Kear-Colwell and Heller (1978); Moenster (1972); Schneider, Gritz, and Jarvik (1975); Taub (1975, 1976); Taub and Kline (1976); Till and Walsh (1980); Whitbourne and Slevin (1978); and Zelinski et al. (1980). The age trends with meaningful verbal material are particularly noteworthy as several authors have suggested that this is the type of memory encountered in daily life in conversations, reading, etc. (Gilbert & Levee, 1971), and that because it is meaningful and close to real experience it maintains a high motivational level across age groups (Hulicka, 1967a; Zelinski et al. 1980).

It therefore seems clear that the age-associated decline in memory performance is not simply a consequence of one particular type of stimulus material being used in the experimental tasks. There have been a few reports that the age trend, while still present, is not as dramatic when the material is presented auditorially, rather than visually (e.g., Arenberg, 1968b; McGhie, Chapman, & Lawson, 1965), but even these claims have been disputed in other reports (e.g., Arenberg, 1976; Craik, 1968; Talland, 1968; Taub, 1972, 1975, 1976). We will see that age trends in memory performance differ as a function of several variables, but it does not appear that stimulus type or stimulus modality are among those variables.

Localizing the Loss

Much of the research investigating memory during adulthood has been conducted with the goal of identifying the specific memory processes or mechanisms that are most affected by increased age. In the pursuit of this localization or isolation strategy, most researchers have employed one or more of the conceptualizations of memory in vogue at that time. The field of memory has been a source of active theoretical speculation and consequently there has been no lack of conceptualizations to help guide research. Many of these models have influenced research on aging, but only four or five have had a substantial impact. In the remainder of this chapter we will examine these ways of conceptualizing memory, and the age trends observed in the postulated mechanisms, in approximate chronological order of their introduction into research on aging.

Interference

A number of researchers have made vague reference to the concept of interference in attempting to "explain" age differences in memory functioning. Precisely what has been meant by this term has never been clearly stated, but it appears to have been used in at least three different ways.

Unfamiliarity. One of the earliest usages of the interference concept was by Ruch (1934) in the context of the disruption (or interference) of habitual associations by new arrangements or relationships among items. Ruch hypothesized that new, unfamiliar associations should be particularly difficult to form in the older nervous system already set with established associations. Essentially, then, Ruch was suggesting that unfamiliar material, that which was not in accord with previous learning, would be more interfering for older individuals than familiar material. Ruch (1934) found some support for this hypothesis in that paired-associate learning of familiar material (highly associated words) exhibited smaller age differences than less familiar material (incorrect mathematical equations). These results were later confirmed by Korchin and Basowitz (1957) using the same types of material.

Subsequent research in this area has relied on normative values of the association strength between the stimulus and response terms in paired-associate learning as the index of preexperimental familiarity. These association-strength norms are obtained by presenting stimulus words to large numbers of individuals with instructions to produce immediate associations of the word, and then recording the number of individuals producing each association. The more people that give a particular word as an association to the stimulus, the higher the associative strength of the response word to the stimulus word. The results from studies manipulating associative strength in this manner have been quite consistent in demonstrating a greater age impairment with items of low associative strength compared to items of high associative strength (e.g., Botwinick & Storandt, 1974a; Canestrari, 1966; Kausler & Lair, 1966; Lair, Moon, & Kausler, 1969; Ross, 1968; Shaps & Nilsson, 1980; Zaretsky & Halberstam, 1968).

The consistency of the above result indicates that one can be fairly confident that the magnitude of age differences are related to stimulus familiarity. What this means, however, is still not clear. It may be the case that unfamiliar material is more interfering with already established neural associations, as Ruch had suggested. On the other hand, in all of the studies cited above it could be argued that the familiarity manipulation was con-founded with level of difficulty. As the material was made less familiar and more interfering with past experience, it also became more difficult for individuals of all ages and thus the relatively greater impairment of older adults may be due to the increased difficulty, rather than the "interfering" nature, of the material. At the present time it does not appear possible to disentangle these two issues, and thus no definite conclusion can be reached about the unfamiliarity aspect of interference as a factor contributing to age differences in memory performance.

A related issue concerns the possibility of generational differences in familiarity with the material often used in memory research. It has been reported that the word-association norms changed from 1927 to 1954 (Jenkins & Russell, 1960), and although recent investigations failed to find any noteworthy age differences in other characteristics of verbal stimuli (e.g., Howard, 1980; Kausler, 1980), it is possible that some age differences in memory might be attributable to age differences in item familiarity. This hypothesis has been the subject of at least five published investigations, but the results have been mixed and no conclusion is yet possible. Howell (1972) compared memory for pictures of contemporary objects and for pictures of "dated" objects from the 1908 Sears catalog, and found smaller age differences with the "dated" material. Poon and Fozard (1978), employing similar material, actually found that older adults (ages 60–70 years) were faster and slightly more accurate at identifying the "dated" objects than were young (ages 18–22 years) adults. Barrett and Wright (1981) contrasted "young words" (e.g., bummer, freon, cassette) with "old words" (e.g., poultice, settee, teacakes) in young (mean age 21 years) and old (mean age 70 years) adults, and found that each group performed best with their "age-appropriate" material. One can question the relevance of each of these findings to contemporary studies of memory and aging, however, since almost no research is done with such markedly biased material.

Two studies using a paired-associate task appear to address the issue of differential stimulus familiarity more directly. Winn, Elias, and Marshall (1976) contrasted young and old adults in the learning of lists with material from 1928 or 1960 norms, and Wittels (1972) compared young (mean age 20 years) and old (mean age 71 years) adults in the learning of lists with associates generated by another person of one's own age or by a person in the other (young or old) age group. Both studies found young individuals to be superior to old ones with each type of material. This finding suggests that any differences in the associative strength of items across age groups are probably not large enough to be responsible for more than a very small proportion of the age differences typically observed in paired-associate performance.

Concurrent Activity. A second manner in which the concept of interference has been invoked to account for age differences in memory refers to the impairment produced by the requirement to perform some other activity while simultaneously attempting to remember information. Welford (1958) summarized much early work on age and skill (including memory), and interpreted it as reflecting an age change in the susceptibility to interference by concurrent activity. For example, Welford described an experiment by Kay in which the performance of older adults was greatly affected by increasing the number of items to be remembered while monitoring a display, but the performance of younger adults was either not affected or only slightly affected.

A great deal of research can be assembled in support of this interference-susceptibility hypothesis. For example, Kirchner (1958), Brinley and Fichter (1970), Botwinick and Storandt (1974a), and Wright (1981) have reported variations of Kay's experiment with the same basic result—age differences increase with the memory demands of the concurrent activity. Gilbert (1941) and Bromley (1958), but not Botwinick and Storandt (1974a), have also reported that older adults suffer more than young adults when required to reorganize the input sequence in a digit-span task and to repeat the items in the reverse order from that in which they were initially presented. Further, Talland (1965) found a greater age-associated decline in a recall task which required simultaneous retention and reorganization of the material compared to one that merely required retention.

There is also a large and fairly consistent body of literature indicating that age deficits are particularly pronounced in dichotic-listening tasks in which different material is presented simultaneously to the two ears. Some of the studies report that age differences only occur in the performance of the material recalled second (e.g., Caird, 1966; Inglis & Ankus, 1965; Inglis, Ankus, & Sykes, 1968; Inglis & Caird, 1963; MacKay & Inglis, 1963; Parkinson, Lindholm, & Urell, 1980), while others report age differences in both the first and the second recalled set (e.g., Clark & Knowles, 1973; Craik, 1965; Inglis & Tansey, 1967; Schonfield, Trueman & Kline, 1972), but all are similar in indicating that the dichotic-listening task is particularly sensitive to the effects of aging. Broadbent and Gregory (1965) and McGhie et al. (1965) have also demonstrated that simultaneous visual and auditory presentations, rather than two simultaneous auditory presentations, result in comparable age deficits.

As was the case with the unfamiliarity aspect of interference, however, it could be argued that in all of these studies task difficulty is inextricably confounded with the requirement to perform some other activity. When a task demands that one's attention be divided among two or more activities, it not only involves the possibility of concurrent interference, but it also becomes more difficult. It therefore seems that the interference-susceptiblity interpretation cannot yet be evaluated independent of the level of difficulty.

Prior or Subsequent Activity. The third major way in which interference has been introduced in research on memory and aging is the manner in which the concept has been used in traditional verbal-learning research. Here there is no confounding with level of difficulty as acquisition and retention on the same primary task is evaluated as a function of the amount and type of prior (proactive interference), or subsequent (retroactive interference), learning.

Although not formally stated, the implicit arguments in this type of interpretation are that because the older individual has accumulated more prior memories, there is greater competition in memory for the storage of new information. An early anecdote illustrating the displacement aspect of this type of interference describes a professor of ichythyology who, upon becoming a dean of students, complained that everytime he learned the name of a new student he forgot the name of another fish. The major assumption in this type of interpretation, therefore, is that memory is finite and that once the storage limit is reached, new information can be retained only by displacing old information.

The ideal procedure for assessing the magnitude of proactive inhibition or interference involves examining performance on a given learning or memory task after various amounts of prior learning. In most situations, however, the proactive-interference comparisons are made with different lists of material, and each successive list is assumed to be contributing to the accumulation of proactive interference. Five aging studies have been reported in which performance decline over progressive lists has been systematically examined, and in four it was found that the rate of proactive-interference accumulation was very similar in groups of young and old adults (Craik, 1968; Elias & Hirasuna, 1976; Fozard & Waugh, 1969; Mistler-Lachman, 1977; but not Hartley & Walsh, 1980). That is, younger adults generally had higher memory scores than older adults, but both groups had nearly equivalent declines across successive lists. A tentative conclusion, then, is that susceptibility to proactive interference does not appear to differ across the adult life span.

An optimum design for assessing retroactive-interference effects involves comparing initial and subsequent acquisition of the same information when the interval between the two tests is filled with learning material of different levels of similarity to the original material, or is filled with different amounts of interpolated activity.

A major limitation with much of the aging research in retroactive interference is that there are typically age differences in initial acquisition that produce serious problems for all later comparisons. If the task is presented for a fixed number of trials the older adult will likely have a lower degree of initial and/or interpolated learning. On the other hand, if the tasks are learned to the same criterion the older adults are likely to require more trials for acquisition and thus will have more total exposure to the initial and/or interpolated material. Attempting to solve this problem by using a statistical adjustment (e.g., analysis of covariance) to control for differences in initial learning, as was done in several studies (e.g., Arenberg, 1967a; Gladis & Braun, 1958; Wimer & Wigdor, 1958), is not appropriate because the age group effect may also be eliminated with this adjustment (Evans & Anastasio, 1968; Storandt & Hudson, 1975).

One basis for comparison of retroactive-interference effects is to examine performance as the percentage savings in relearning relative to original learning after different types of retention-interval activity. Alternatively, one could examine the percentage of items correctly recalled on the first relearning trial in the control (no interpolated activity) and experimental (interpolated interfering activity) condition. In three separate experiments allowing one or both of these types of comparisons (i.e., Hulicka, 1967b; Traxler, 1973; Wimer & Wigdor, 1958) there was no consistent age trend in the magnitude of the interference effect. These methods of comparison are also flawed, because there is no control of degree of exposure to the interpolated material, but it is clear that there is not yet any convincing evidence of age differences in retroactive-interference susceptibility with existing procedures.

Another comparison relevant to the issue of amount of retroactive interference in various age groups was reported by Smith (1974, 1975a), who compared the functions relating recall accuracy to recall output position. He found that the slopes of these interference functions were not significantly different across three age groups, thus suggesting that increased age is not associated with greater susceptibility to interference from previous responses.

A later experiment by the same author, Smith (1979), also found no evidence for age differences in the effects of retroactive interference. Young (ages 20–39 years), middle-aged (ages 40–59 years), and old (ages 60–80 years) adults received lists of words with the instructions to recall items after the last word in a given list from the list prior to the one just presented. Amount of retroactive interference was assessed by comparing recall performance when the intervening list contained 10, 20, or 40 items. As expected, performance decreased with a greater number of intervening items, but the rate of decrease was nearly identical across the three age groups. The implication of this result is that susceptibility to retroactive interference apparently does not differ across the adult life span.

On the basis of the evidence reviewed above it does not appear that the interference hypothesis, in any of its three versions, provides a very satisfactory explanation of adult age differences in memory. Interference viewed as unfamiliarity or concurrent activity is confounded with task difficulty, and the existence of greater age differences under "interfering" conditions might simply be attributable to a general tendency for age impairments to be proportional to task demands. Methodological problems hamper the interpretation of studies investigating amount of proactive and retroactive interference in various age groups, although there appear to be little or no age differences in susceptibility to either proactive or retroactive interference.

Memory Stages

Another conceptualization of memory that has been useful in guiding research on age differences in memory functioning is based on a trichotomous distinction among registration, retention, and recall, or in more recent terminology, among encoding, storage, and retrieval. Registration or encoding refers to the initial establishment of a neural code of the information, retention or storage refers to the preservation of the information over time, and recall or retrieval refers to the recovery and use of information at the time of testing. Successful memory performance obviously requires each stage to be functional, but unsuccessful memory performance could be due to a problem in one, two, or all three, of the hypothetical stages. The goal of research conducted under this memory stage framework has been to determine the relative importance of each stage for age deficits in memory.

Encoding. One of the most generally accepted conclusions with respect to memory stages is that the encoding stage presents particular problems for older adults.

Imagery. A specific manifestation of this encoding difficulty is evident in the use of visual imagery or other mnemonic techniques to establish meaningful links between the items that are to be remembered, or between those items and more permanent information in long-term memory. Research over the last 10–20 years has clearly established the beneficial effects of such mnemonic tricks as using bizarre imagery, locations, or rhymes to help remember many different types of information. However, a fairly consistent finding in research with adults of different ages is that older adults report the use of mediators much less frequently in their memorizing attempts than younger adults (e.g., Hulicka & Grossman, 1967; Hulicka & Rust, 1964; Hulicka, Sterns, & Grossman, 1967; Hulicka & Weiss, 1965; Rowe & Schnore, 1971).

On the basis of the finding just described, several investigators have attempted to induce older individuals to use mediational strategies to determine whether age differences might be eliminated under facilitating conditions. The results of these studies have been mixed, and it seems likely that methodological factors have been contributing to some of the confusion. For example, Canestrari (1968) found that old adults improved more than young adults with the provision of a mediator, but the task was so easy that the young participants were near perfect in their performance even without mediators and hence they had less room for improvement when the mediator was provided. Hulicka and Grossman (1967) handled the differential-difficulty problem by requiring the young (mean age 16 years) adults to remember a list of 20 words, while the old (mean age 74 years) adults had to remember only 10 words. It was reported that the two age groups achieved comparable proportions of items recalled when a mediator was provided, but since this means that the young participants actually recalled twice as many words as the old participants the exact interpretation of this finding is not clear. Treat and Reese (1976) also reported the elimination of age differences when a mediator was used by all individuals, but they employed an inappropriate covariance adjustment in analyzing the data, and they examined only the data from the first trial in which there was likely very large variability. Providing imagery instructions resulted in greater reduction in the number of trials to a learning criterion for elderly (mean age 73 years) than for young (mean age 22 years) adults in a study by Poon and Walsh-Sweeney (1981), but the differential benefit was apparently transient as it did not persist in subsequent retention tests. Treat, Poon, and Fozard (1981) replicated and extended these results in the finding that older adults exhibited short-term benefit of imagery instructions, but there was no sustained improvement over intervals of two weeks.

Three recent studies without these methodological or consistency problems indicated that the benefit of imagery mediation relative to young adults was greater for middle-aged but not for old adults (Mason & Smith, 1977), was not differentially effective across age groups (Whitbourne & Slevin, 1978), or had slightly greater effect for older adults without eliminating the age differences (Treat, Poon, Fozard, & Popkin, 1978).

In the face of the inconsistency in the results surveyed above it appears impossible to draw a definite conclusion about whether explicit mediational instructions are of any greater help to older adults than to younger ones. In fact, there is some evidence that older adults actually derive less benefit from a mediator than do younger adults. Both Hulicka and Grossman (1967) and Hulicka et al. (1967) have reported data suggesting that when a mediator is used for a pair of words the resulting recall is greater for young adults than for old adults. In an interesting extension of this line of research, Marshall, Elias, Webber, Gist, Winn, and King (1978) found that young people learned faster with mediators generated by other young individuals than with mediators generated by older individuals, although the two sets of mediators were not easily discriminable and had no obvious structural differences. This result might be interpreted as indicating that older adults are not only less effective users of externally provided mediators, but are also less efficient producers of effective mediators.

While much of the experimental research has been inconclusive, the consistency with which older adults report not using mediational processes suggests that ineffective use of imagery and mediation may be contributing to the poorer memory performance of older adults in many laboratory tasks. The possibility that this deficiency can be corrected with instructions or special conditions cannot yet be evaluated because of inadequate data.

Organization. A second aspect of encoding that has been found to exert a substantial influence on the memory performance of young adults is the organization imposed on the material to be remembered. Several lines of research demonstrate that meaningful structuring or organizing of information at the time of presentation generally facilitates recall, but that older adults typically engage in less of this beneficial organization than young adults.

One class of research has found that stimulus material with the most potential for organization exhibits the greatest differences between young and old adults. Heron and Craik (1964), for example, found that young and old individuals matched for memory span with meaningless material (Finnish digits) nevertheless exhibited age differences with more meaningful material (English digits), presumably because the young adults were better able to organize this material than older adults. Craik (1968) and Taub (1974) also found no age differences with unorganizable material (color names or random letters), while young adults were markedly superior with material that could be easily organized (text sentences or letters grouped into words). Greater age differences under conditions most favorable to internal organization have also been reported by Kausler and Puckett (1979), contrasting high frequency words and low frequency words (the former assumed to have more associations that could promote organization), and Laurence and Trotter (1971), contrasting blocked and random arrangement of related words (the former presumably facilitating organization according to meaning).

The evidence on this issue is not entirely consistent as one manipulation has produced contradictory results. Craik and Masani (1967) systematically varied the closeness with which strings of words approximated meaningful English sentences and found that young adults improved more than old adults in recall performance as the approximation to English increased. A later attempt at replicating this finding (Craik & Masani, 1969) failed to reveal any differential age effects, however, and a similar study by Kinsbourne (1973) also failed to find any age differences in the effect of variations in approximation to English on recall performance. These exceptions are puzzling, but the weight of the evidence seems to favor the view that age differences are accentuated when the conditions are most favorable for organization.

In a related vein, three studies (Friedman, 1966, 1974; Kinsbourne, 1973) have reported that the performance differences between young and old adults are larger when the recall is scored with respect to the exact order of presentation compared to when free (unordered) recall is allowed. One interpretation of this result is that the requirement of maintaining the original organization of the material presents a special difficulty for older individuals.

A number of experimenters have attempted to discover evidence for age differences in organizational processes by analyzing the recall protocols of participants, but the attempts have met with varied success. Laurence (1966) and Hultsch (1971a) found no age differences in the consistency of recall order over trials, an index which is presumed to reflect the internal organization of the material. Using a measure of recall clustering according to the semantic relationships of the randomly presented items, which indicates the amount of internal reorganization of the material, Eysenck (1974), Gordon (1975), and Howard et al. (1981) reported no significant age differences between young and old adults. However Denney (1974) found that middle-aged individuals (ages 30–60 years) exhibited more clustering than old individuals (ages 70–90 years) and Horn et al. (1981) found organization measures to be negatively correlated with increased age. Sanders et al. (1980) also reported that young adults (mean age 24 years) clustered more and exhibited evidence of greater organization while rehearsing than older adults (mean age 74 years).

Hultsch (1974) has argued that some of these measures of organization are unfairly biased against young adults since they fail to account for more rapid improvement in performance of young adults compared to older adults across successive trials. With alternative measures of input-output and output-output consistency, Hultsch (1974) did find that increased age (range 18–85 years) was negatively associated with measures of mnemonic organization. Smith (1980) confirmed this finding and also demonstrated that younger adults do indeed exhibit greater increases in organization across successive trials.

At the present time it is perhaps best to reserve judgment with respect to whether age differences are evident in measures of organization derived from recall protocols. The available evidence is still too inconsistent to warrant any reasonably definitive conclusion.

Only slightly more confidence can be attached to conclusions based on deliberate attempts to encourage organization through manipulations of instructions or presentation conditions. Hultsch (1971b) found that the age difference in recall between young (ages 20–29 years) and middle-aged (ages 40–49 years) adults was eliminated by the requirement to sort the items to be remembered into categories before the recall test. Smith (1977) also reported that age differences among young, middle, and old groups were eliminated by presenting semantic cues with each item at the initial presentation; a manipulation that presumably increased the organizational potential of the items. Deliberate instructions to organize the items during presentation did not lead to significantly greater effects in older adults in a study by Hultsch (1969), although there was a tendency for older individuals of low verbal ability to exhibit greater performance increases than younger, low-verbal-ability individuals.

A reasonable conclusion with respect to aging and organizational processes in memory is that older adults engage less frequently, and perhaps less successfully, in the types of organization that facilitate memory performance. No one source of evidence is completely compelling, but the consistency with which age differences in organization are reported makes it quite likely that a real difference in organization exists.

Pacing. Another rather dramatic example of an age deficit in the encoding stage is the finding that the magnitude of age differences in learning, memory, and comprehension tasks tends to decrease when the rate of stimulus presentation is slower (e.g., Adamowicz, 1976; Arenberg, 1965; 1967b; Canestrari, 1963; Cohen, 1979; Eisdorfer, Axelrod, & Wilkie, 1963; Kinsbourne, 1973; Kinsbourne & Berryhill, 1972; Taub, 1967). There are some exceptions to this finding (e.g., Mason & Smith, 1977; Monge & Hultsch, 1971; Smith, 1976; Taub, 1966; 1968), but it is more often the case that the less time allowed for stimulus encoding the greater the age differences that result in subsequent tests of memory. This, of course, is indirect evidence, but it is certainly consistent with the interpretation that older individuals have particular problems with the encoding stage of memory.

Possible Mechanism. An intriguing speculation as to a mechanism responsible for the problem of older adults in the encoding stage has been offered by Perlmutter (1978, 1979b). Noting that previous researchers have reported that there is greater variability in word associates produced by older adults than by young adults (e.g., Riegel & Birren, 1965; Riegel & Riegel, 1964; Tresselt & Mayzner, 1964), Perlmutter suggested that encoding inconsistency could be responsible for some of the observed memory deficits. Older adults might be more variable in their encodings of an identical stimulus across time, and thus would be less likely to generate the same encoding during the acquisition and test phases. Perlmutter (1979b) reported a study investigating this encoding-variability hypothesis, and did find that the older individuals produced fewer repetitions of word associations on successive trials than younger individuals. The task instructions were quite vague, however, and it may be that the differences were more a reflection of personal style rather than actual capability.

A similar mechanism, but operating in the opposite direction, was postulated by Simon and Craik (described in Craik and Simon, 1980). The task in this experiment was cued recall of words originally presented in sentences. Two types of cues were used; context-specific, consisting of the adjective preceding the word in the sentence, and general, consisting of a simple definition of the word. The "young" and "old" groups (no details about ages or sample sizes were provided) were found to have equivalent recall performance with the general cues, but the young were better and the old were worse with the context-specific cues. Craik and Simon (1980) suggested that older adults might "have a tendency to be less influenced by the context, to encode events in a similar way from occasion to occasion . . ." (p. 106). In other words, age-associated memory problems might be a consequence of encodings that are too stereotyped, rather than too variable.

Although the Perlmutter and Simon and Craik interpretations are in a sense contradictory, both rely on the notion of encoding specificity as a factor in the memory problems of older adults. It therefore seems likely that further research in this area would prove informative. At the present time the speculations must be considered interesting and provocative, but by no means verified.

Storage. Age-related problems in storage have been rather difficult to investigate because of the known (or suspected) age differences in acquisition. If older individuals never acquired the material to the same degree as younger ones, it is impossible to attribute subsequent recall failures to a problem of storage. Fortunately there have been several techniques developed that allow a way around this difficulty.

Equating for Acquisition. One of these techniques is to examine retention only after individuals in different age groups have been equated for level of acquisition. This should not be a statistical adjustment of initial acquisition because of problems with analysis-of-covariance techniques when the covariate is correlated with the independent variable (e.g., Evans & Anastasio, 1968; Storandt & Hudson, 1975), but rather all individuals should be taken to the same criterion of initial learning. Recall or relearning performance can then be compared as a relatively "pure" measure of retention.

Two studies using this "equating for acquisition" technique (Desroches, Kaiman, & Ballard, 1966; Hulicka, 1965) did not find age differences in the rate of initial learning, perhaps because middle-aged rather than young adults were used (i.e., individuals aged 30–39 years in the Hulicka study, and with a mean age of 45 years in the Desroches et al. study). These studies should probably be ignored, therefore, since it is difficult to interpret retention findings when the samples of adults were apparently not typical, as judged by the absence of expected age differences in rate of initial learning.

The remaining studies are fairly consistent when the interval between acquisition and test is considered. Three experiments (Hulicka & Rust, 1964; Hulicka & Weiss, 1965; Wimer & Wigdor, 1958) found no age differences with retention intervals of 15–20 minutes; two studies (Wimer, 1960b; Hulicka & Rust, 1964) found an age impairment with a 24-hour interval; and four of five studies (Belbin & Downs, 1964, 1965; Harwood & Naylor, 1969; Hulicka & Rust, 1964; but not Hulicka & Weiss, 1965) found age differences at retention intervals of three days to one month. Poon and Walsh-Sweeney (1981) examined retention of perfectly learned paired-associates after intervals of 45 minutes, 1 day, 1 week, and 1 month, and found progressively greater age differences in favor of the young adults with increasing interval. Taken together, these studies seem to suggest that there is no age deficit in short-term storage over 15–30 minutes, but that older individuals may suffer more than young ones with intervals greater than 24 hours.

Rate of Forgetting. A second technique for investigating age differences in storage makes no attempt to equate the level of acquisition but instead examines the relationship between memory accuracy and interval since initial acquisition. If information is lost from storage at a faster rate in older adults, the function relating memory performance to retention interval should exhibit a steeper drop for them than for younger adults. However, if individuals of all age groups lose information from storage at the same rate then the functions should be parallel.

One task in which this "rate of forgetting" comparison has been examined is a recognition procedure in which a series of items is presented with the participant asked to decide whether specific probe items were presented earlier in the list. The general finding is that accuracy of identifying an item as old or new decreases with the number of items (i.e., with time, since items are usually presented at a fixed rate) intervening between the initial presentation and the occurrence of the probe item. Of particular relevance to the present argument is that at least six independent studies have reported that although the initial level of accuracy is often lower with increased age, the rate of decline for intervals greater than about 10 seconds is almost identical across adult age groups (e.g., Craik, 1969, 1971; Erber, 1978; Ferris et al. 1980; Poon & Fozard, 1980; Wickelgren, 1975).

Talland (1968) employed a running-span version of this procedure in which accuracy was assessed for items at varying positions from the end of lists of different lengths. Data from two experiments with 36 and 40 individuals per

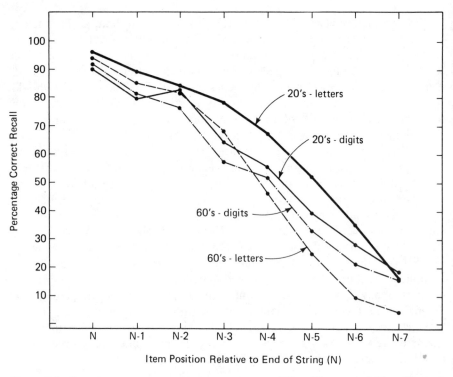

Figure 7.3. Running memory span in two age groups (20 to 29 years and 60 to 69 years) for letter and digit material. Data from Talland (1968).

decade are illustrated in Figure 7.3. Notice that the functions relating recall accuracy to item position are quite parallel across age groups. This can be interpreted as indicating that the rate at which items are lost from memory is approximately the same across age groups.

A very similar finding of parallel forgetting functions has also been reported in tasks where several items are presented, a retention interval is filled with some type of distracting activity, and then an attempt is made to recall the original items. Most studies of this type have found that recall accuracy declines with the length of the retention interval, and four studies have indicated that the rate of decline is no greater for old individuals than for young ones (i.e., Keevil-Rogers & Schnore, 1969; Kriauciunas, 1968; Schonfield, 1972; Talland, 1967). Three types of tasks utilizing the rate-of-forgetting technique are therefore consistent in indicating that regardless of the level of initial acquisition, the proportion of information that is preserved over time is approximately the same in adults of all ages.

Cumulative Learning. The third technique that has been employed to investigate possible age differences in storage is almost the converse of the rate-of-forgetting technique. This is an indirect procedure in which the cumulative learning of repeated presentations of the same item is examined. The reasoning is that the rate of learning should be slower if less information is preserved from one presentation to the next, but that learning rates should be the same if there are no differences in the amount of information retained. In order to minimize the use of conscious learning strategies that could lead to encoding differences the participants should be unaware of the repetition of the items. This can be done by presenting lists of meaningless letters or digits with, for example, every third list being repeated. Of the five experiments that have been reported using this technique, four (Caird, 1966; Heron & Craik, 1964, Exps. II and III; Talland, 1968) reported no age differences in the rate of cumulative learning, while one (Heron & Craik, 1964, Exp. I) found that young adults improved with repetitions whereas older adults did not.

On the basis of very similar findings with the "equating for acquisition," "rate of forgetting," and "cumulative learning" techniques, we can be fairly confident that age differences in the storage stage of memory are slight to nonexistent. This conclusion must be qualified somewhat, however, since all of the evidence indicating no age differences in storage processes dealt with time intervals of less than 30 minutes and there is some indication that older adults might be impaired with intervals of 24 hours or more.

Retrieval. Many researchers have argued that the retrieval stage is a source of particular difficulty for older adults, but a close examination of the evidence indicates that this conclusion is still rather equivocal.

Recall versus Recognition. One of the major arguments implicating a retrieval problem in older age is based on the different pattern of results sometimes obtained on recognition tests of memory compared to recall tests. It is assumed that if an item can be recognized as one previously presented then it must have been encoded and stored. However, if the item cannot be recalled but can be recognized, one might infer that the difficulty was in retrieval since recall tests presumably require more of a retrieval component than do recognition tests.

There are at least three problems with this argument. The first is that the empirical findings are not nearly as consistent as implied by the early advocates of this position. Several studies have reported no significant age differences in recognition performance (e.g., Craik, 1969, 1971; Kausler, Kleim, & Overcast, 1975; McCormack, 1982, Exp. 2; Schonfield, 1965; Schonfield & Robertson, 1966; Shaps & Nilsson, 1980; Smith, 1975b), but even more studies have reported moderate to large age differences (e.g., Botwinick & Storandt, 1974a; Bruning, Holzbauer, & Kimberlin 1975; Cerella et al., 1982; Erber, 1974, 1978; Fozard & Waugh, 1969; Fullerton & Smith, 1980; Gordon & Clark, 1974a, 1974b; Harkins, Chapman, & Eisdorfer, 1979; Harwood & Naylor, 1969; Kausler & Kleim, 1978; Kausler & Puckett, 1981a; McCormack, 1981, 1982, Exp. 1; Perlmutter, 1978; Rankin & Kausler, 1979; Schonfield et al., 1972; Wickelgren, 1975; Witte & Freund, 1976; Zelinski et al. 1980).

The second problem is that it is by no means established that the primary difference between recognition and recall is that the latter involves retrieval and the former does not. In fact, a phenomenon known as recognition failure suggests that this distinction is erroneous, or at best, incomplete. Tulving and Thomson (1973) demonstrated that if individuals learn words in the context of other strongly associated words, they will sometimes fail to recognize the critical words in a recognition test but will be able to recall them if cued with the strong associate. Recall without recognition should be impossible if the only difference between the two is that recall involves retrieval whereas recognition does not. The existence of recognition failure followed by successful cued recall has now been documented in several studies, including at least one involving older adults (i.e., Shaps & Nilsson, 1980), and thus the recognition-recall distinction on the basis of retrieval demands is in considerable doubt.

Another problem with this argument is that recognition tasks are also generally easier than recall tasks, and therefore the degree of retrieval in a recognition-recall contrast is confounded with the level of difficulty (see Botwinick, 1978; McNulty & Caird, 1966). Thus, between-task comparisons are not meaningful unless there is some independent assurance that the various tasks are of equivalent difficulty. At the present time, it simply is not possible to determine whether older adults are at a greater disadvantage in recall tasks than in recognition tasks because the former have a greater retrieval component than the latter, or because the former are more difficult than the latter.

Cued Recall. A similar argument concerning the confounding of type of task with level of difficulty applies to a second body of evidence often cited as indicative of a retrieval problem in older adults. Laurence (1967) reported that older (mean age 75 years) adults improved more than young (mean age 20 years) adults when semantic cues about the item's identity were provided at the time of recall. This contrast between free or uncued recall and cued recall has been considered to reflect a difference in the amount of retrieval cues present at the time of recall, but it also could represent a difference in the level of difficulty. A cued-recall test must necessarily be easier than the uncued test, or else one would conclude that the cues were ineffective in facilitating retrieval.

Laurence's (1967) results have also proven difficult to replicate under slightly different conditions. For example, Drachman and Leavitt (1972) found no age difference in the effectiveness of a structural (i.e., first letter of the word) cue, and Smith (1977) found that when the cues were present only at recall there were no age differences in the effectiveness of either structural or semantic (i.e., the taxonomic category of the word) cues. Smith did report that the age differences were eliminated when the semantic cues were available during the initial presentation of the items regardless of whether they were available at the time of recall, but in this case it seems that encoding rather than retrieval processes are involved. Ceci and Tabor (1981) reported a very similar experiment and also found that age differences were eliminated when cues about the taxonomic or thematic grouping of the items were available at both initial presentation and time of recall. A structural cue was found to be equally beneficial to young and old adults by Simon (1979), although the older adults in her experiments derived less benefit from the semantic (synonym) cue. Older adults were actually hindered, whereas young adults were facilitated, by the presence of a semantic (implicational cue) in a study by Till and Walsh (1980). Hultsch (1975) also reported no age difference in the effectiveness of a semantic (category name) cue at recall for the number of words recalled, although he found that the older adults were helped more than the young adults in a measure of the number of words from different categories that were recalled. This latter measure must be viewed with some caution, however, since given a category name it is very easy to think of a common exemplar and thus there may be little or no actual memory involved with this measure.

The situation with respect to the uncued-cued recall comparison is therefore very similar to that with the recognition-recall comparisons, namely, it may be the presumed retrieval requirement or it may be the level of difficulty that distinguishes the tasks. In either case the age patterns are not very consistent and thus it is probably best not to attempt any conclusions from this research at the present time.

Other Evidence. Several other arguments have been proposed in favor of a retrieval deficit in older individuals but none are particularly compelling. For example, a number of researchers have suggested that the age decline in the number of higher-order groupings of items in free-recall tasks (e.g., Craik & Masani, 1967, 1969; Eysenck, 1974; Hultsch, 1975) reflects a deficit in retrieval efficiency. However, it is almost inevitable that when there is a decrease in the number of total words recalled, there will be a similar decrease in the number of higher-order groupings that are recalled. Under these circumstances it does not seem reasonable to claim that the number of groupings accurately reflects efficiency of retrieval.

Craik (1968) has also suggested that retrieval problems become especially pronounced when the number of items in a list is increased, and with his finding that age differences increase with list size he concluded that retrieval processes are impaired with aging. Smith (1979), however, found the exact opposite result, with age differences decreasing as the size of the list increased.

A final argument is based on a small pilot project by Buschke (1974). No statistical evaluation was conducted, but it was reported that middle-aged adults were somewhat less consistent in recalling items over successive recall attempts than were young college students. This finding, if confirmed in a formal investigation, might be interpreted as indicating that the information had been stored but that the effectiveness or consistency of retrieval decreased with age. With the little evidence presently available, however, it is impossible to draw any conclusions from this method.

Despite the general opinion that retrieval represents a special problem for older individuals, it is difficult to identify any definite evidence in support of that position. What is often considered to be the strongest evidence (i.e., the recognition-recall and cued recall-uncued recall contrasts) is confounded with level of difficulty and is not entirely consistent across several published studies. No strong conclusion about retrieval as a major source of age difficulties in memory can therefore be reached at this time.

One reason for the apparent difficulty in isolating the effects of the retrieval stage is that the ease or efficiency of retrieval clearly depends upon the nature of the encoding. Just as the retrievability of documents from one's office depends upon the manner in which they were initially organized and filed, so does the retrieval of items in memory depend upon the type of encoding the items initially received. A growing awareness of the intrinsic interrelationships of encoding, storage, and retrieval processes has led to questions about the appropriateness of this distinction in memory research. If the distinction itself is in doubt, it is unlikely that an approach based upon this distinction will prove very useful in the identification of the factors involved in memory problems associated with increased age.

Memory Stores

A very popular approach to understanding memory involves making distinctions among different types of memory storage systems, either in terms of temporal parameters or functional properties. The categorization of this type that has had the greatest impact in research on adult development distinguishes between primary memory on the one hand, and secondary memory on the other. Primary memory is thought to be a temporary holding or organizing buffer through which all information that will be subsequently remembered must pass. It is roughly analogous to the span of consciousness in that it refers to the information that is in one's immediate awareness or occupies one's current attention. Information is assumed to be maintained in primary memory only by the active process of attention or rehearsal; without such attention the information decays or is displaced from primary memory. Secondary memory in this scheme refers to all of the durable knowledge that one possesses that is not in immediate consciousness. Information in secondary memory does not require active attention for its maintenance, nor is the storage capacity narrowly limited as is the case for primary memory.

The manner in which the primary memory-secondary memory distinction has been used in aging research has been to assume that sizable age differences are present in secondary memory (because most information that is recalled is not recalled directly from immediate consciousness), and then to determine whether age deficits are also present in primary memory.

Measuring Primary Memory. One argument against an age decline in primary memory capacity assumes that immediate memory span is largely determined by primary memory capacity, and since there are very slight differences in memory span across adulthood (cf. Figure 7.2), there must be little or no change in primary memory capacity. While this reasoning is compelling, it is somewhat circular and one would feel more comfortable about the conclusion if independent methods of assessing primary memory could be shown to produce the same result. Unfortunately, the other techniques for assessing primary memory have yielded rather inconsistent results.

Craik (1968) proposed a mathematical technique for estimating primary memory size based on the relationship between recall performance and the number of items to be remembered. With three types of material there was no significant difference between the primary memory estimates of young (mean age 22 years) and old (mean age 65 years) adults, but with the fourth type of material (unrelated words) the estimated capacity of primary memory was larger for young adults than for older adults.

Another technique used to measure primary memory capacity involves presenting a list of 12–30 items for free recall, and then examining the level of recall for the last 3–5 items in the list. The reasoning is that the most recently presented items should still be in immediate consciousness, and thus recall accuracy for those items can serve as an estimate of primary memory functioning. Two early studies (Craik, 1968; Raymond, 1971) employing this technique reported no age differences in primary memory effectiveness, but one of these studies (Raymond, 1971) did not include an appropriate group of young adults and so the results from that study are not very meaningful. Moreover, two later studies (Arenberg, 1976; Salthouse, 1980) found statistically significant age differences in these primary memory measures, with younger individuals scoring higher than older individuals. Robertson-Tchabo and Arenberg (1976) also reported that this measure of primary memory correlates −.24 with age, i.e., the capacity estimates decrease with age between a range of 20 and 80 years. A correlation of −.15 was reported by Horn et al. (1981) in a sample of 105 males between the ages of 20 and 60. Furthermore, two studies by Walsh and his colleagues (Walsh & Baldwin, 1977; Walsh et al. 1980) noted that younger adults had higher estimated primary memory capacities than older adults, i.e., 3.7 versus 3.2 and 3.5 versus 2.9, although in neither case was the age difference statistically significant.

A continuous-recognition task was used by Poon and Fozard (1980) to argue that age differences are more pronounced in secondary than in primary memory. Indeed, these investigators did find a smaller age difference in recognition accuracy when the interval between presentation and test was short and performance was presumably based on primary memory, than when it was long and performance was presumably based on secondary memory. Similarly, Smith (1975a) found very small age differences with short intervals between input and recall, but much larger differences with greater intervals. It is important to note that in both of these cases it is the time in memory rather than some functional property that has been used to distinguish between primary and secondary memory. Whether this is an acceptable means of defining primary memory is still a matter of some dispute.

Hartley and Walsh (1980) examined three alternative measures of primary memory in two groups of adults (mean ages 21 and 69 years). One measure was the number of items recalled in the first 15 seconds of recall, another was the number of words from the last four input positions recalled in the first four output positions, and the third was the number of words from the last four input positions recalled in the first 15 seconds of recall. The measures varied considerably for both age groups (i.e., means of 6.4, 1.4, and 1.7 for young adults, and 4.3, 1.2, and 1.3 for old adults, respectively), and only the first measure yielded statistically significant age differences. As the authors point out, however, "For both age groups the number of recency items appearing in the early stages of recall was well below even a conservative estimate of the capacity of primary memory for words; therefore, we cannot be certain that primary memory did not differ" (p. 903).

A similar state of confusion exists with respect to the primary memory estimates available in data originally reported by Salthouse (1980) and later reanalyzed by Wright (1982). If, following Watkins (1974), primary memory is "defined as the mechanism underyling the recency effect in free recall," one can measure primary memory either by the level of recall of the last four input items (Tulving & Patterson, 1968), or by the level of recall with fewer than seven items intervening between presentation and test (Tulving & Colotla, 1970). Unfortunately, contradictory results were obtained with the two techniques as age differences were pronounced in the first measure, but much smaller and not statistically significant for the second measure.

It is not yet clear whether the absence of age differences with some measures of primary memory is attributable to large variability producing weak statistical tests, or whether there are truly no differences across age groups in this hypothesized process. What is clear, however, is that the currently available measures yield contradictory results and thus it is possible for researchers to espouse either an age-stable or an age-decline position with respect to primary memory functioning by judicious selection of dependent measures.

Based on the research described above it appears that the primary memory-secondary memory distinction has not yet been particularly useful in aging research. The evidence as to the intactness of primary memory throughout the life span is still not very convincing, and if both hypothetical storage systems reveal age declines the distinction will not be very helpful in identifying the specific aspects of memory that are, and are not, age sensitive.

Processing Depth

A relatively recent interpretation of memory functioning focuses on the depth of processing the to-be-remembered information. A fundamental assumption is that incoming stimuli are subjected to different amounts of initial processing and, other things being equal, those stimuli receiving the "deepest" levels of processing (i.e., semantic or conceptual rather than sensory or structural) will have the most durable and strongest memory representations. As applied to aging, this perspective maintains that older adults either do not, or cannot, engage in the "deep" levels of processing that are responsible for superior memory performance.

Orienting Tasks. One of the most popular procedures for investigating the effect of levels of processing in memory is to instruct the participants to perform various orienting tasks during the initial presentation of the items, and then to examine performance across conditions in a subsequent memory test. Shallow levels of processing are produced by requesting judgments about superficial characteristics (e.g., how many letters are in this word?), while deep processing is produced by requesting conceptual or semantic judgments (e.g., what is a synonym of this word?). The results with this orienting-task procedure in studies with adults of varying ages have been mixed. Several studies have reported that older adults are apparently less capable of deep processing as age differences in recall were found to be largest under conditions that involved the deepest levels of processing (Erber, Herman, & Botwinick, 1980; Eysenck, 1974; Mason, 1979; Simon, 1979; White, described in Craik, 1977). However, two studies employing recognition measures yielded results in contradiction to one another (Mason, 1979; White, described in Craik, 1977), and a third (Erber et al., 1980) obtained inconclusive results (i.e., an age by depth interaction at $p < .07$). Moreover, three recent studies with recall measures (Craik, described in Craik and Simon, 1980; Till & Walsh, 1980; Zelinski, Walsh, & Thompson, 1978) and two with recognition measures (Craik, described in Craik & Simon, 1980; Smith & Winograd, 1978) failed to find significant Age by Depth interactions. (See Burke and Light, 1981, for further discussion of these studies.)

It might also be expected from the processing-depth perspective that, other things being equal, the more different orienting tasks performed on a stimulus the greater the total processing depth associated with that stimulus. Barrett and Wright (1981) examined performance in an unexpected recall test after one or two orienting tasks and found that both young (ages 18–24 years) and old (ages 63–75 years) adults averaged about one additional correct word when there were two orienting tasks rather than just one. The stimulus items in this study were highly unusual words, however, and there was no overall age difference in free-recall performance. Because this is an atypical finding, one must be very cautious in interpreting these results in the context of the processing-depth hypothesis.

False Recognitions. Smith (1975b) and Rankin and Kausler (1979) employed a false-recognition procedure to investigate the processing-depth explanation of adult age differences in memory. This procedure involves the presentation of a series of words with the participant required to select previously presented words in the context of distractors that are similar either superficially (i.e., either visually or acoustically), or semantically (i.e., synonyms), to the old words. Both groups of investigators reported that older adults made more false recognitions of semantically similar distractor items than young adults, but they interpreted their results differently. Smith (1975b, p. 363) concluded that: ". . . the older participants were less able to distinguish the correct alternatives from their semantic distractors because of incomplete semantic processing at the time of presentation," while Rankin and Kausler (1979, p. 63) argued that: "Whatever age-related deficits take place in the encoding of information on a recognition memory task, they do not involve the failure to encode informational inputs either phonologically or semantically."

This conflict illustrates a serious problem with the false-recognition procedure; one attempts to make inferences about the nature of the processing on the basis of the frequency of certain types of errors, but it is not clear whether an increase in a certain type of error signifies more or less of the relevant processing. Smith (1975b) suggested that more errors in the older adults indicated poorer semantic processing, while Rankin and Kausler (1979) appear to argue that more errors indicate equivalent or superior semantic processing among the elderly. In the face of this confusion, and the failure to find any age differences in semantic recognition errors by Coyne, Herman and Botwinick (1980), it is perhaps best to disregard the results from the false-recognition procedure as they pertain to the processing-depth hypothesis.

Incidental Learning. One implication of the processing-depth hypothesis is that the age differences should be smallest on tasks in which the processing depth is the shallowest. That is, to the extent that all individuals process the items superficially, there is little opportunity for the greater processing ability of the younger adults to produce superior performance. An incidental-learning paradigm provides a reasonable test of this implication as participants are tested for the retention of material that they were not specifically instructed to learn.

The orienting-task procedure includes a form of incidental learning since the participants are not informed that they will later be tested for their memory of the items they are classifying. However, as discussed earlier the results from studies using orienting tasks have not been very consistent. Most such studies have reported that age differences are evident in some, but not all, of the incidental learning conditions (e.g., Erber et al., 1980; Eysenck, 1974; Mason, 1979; Till & Walsh, 1980; White, described in Craik, 1977; Zelinski et al., 1978), although two studies found age differences in all incidental conditions (i.e., Craik, described in Craik & Simon, 1980; Smith & Winograd, 1978).

A great variety of other incidental-learning procedures have also been employed, and the results from these procedures have been somewhat more consistent. Four studies found no age differences in incidental-learning performance (Hulicka, 1965; Perlmutter, 1978,; 1979a; Wimer, 1960a), but one of these (Hulicka, 1965) also failed to find age differences in intentional learning and since this is quite unusual the samples may have been atypical. Another

(Wimer, 1960a) employed very small sample sizes (i.e., 10 and 6 individuals in young and old groups, respectively), and the remaining two (Perlmutter, 1978, 1979a) reported that age differences in incidental learning were large and significant with a recall test but were less pronounced and not significant with an easier recognition test. On the other hand, quite a few studies have reported significant age differences with incidental-learning tasks. Thorndike et al. (1928), Willoughby (1929), and Erber (1976) found that older adults were less accurate at retaining the code associations after performing a code-substitution task; Bromley (1958) and Peak (1968) found that older adults recalled fewer names of subtests after performing in a battery of tests; Horn et al. (1981) reported a decrease with increased age in accuracy of reporting details of an incidental event; Kausler and Lair (1965) and Lair et al. (1969) found that older adults recalled fewer backward (i.e., response-stimulus rather than stimulus-response) associations after a paired-associate learning procedure; and Nebes and Andrews-Kulis (1976) and Mergler et al. (1977) found that older adults were poorer at recalling incidental stimulus pairings after performing in a primary task.

The remarkable consistency with which age differences have been reported despite the many different procedures that have been employed dictates a conclusion that, contrary to the predictions from the processing-depth interpretation, older adults are poorer than younger adults with incidental-learning tasks.

The depth-of-processing interpretation is still being actively investigated, but the presently available evidence is not very favorable for this perspective. The results from experiments employing orienting tasks to control depth of processing are not consistent with one another, and the outcomes from the false-recognition procedure are confusing and at least partially contradictory. The greatest consistency noted was in the report of age differences in incidental learning, a finding the opposite of what would be predicted from a processing-depth age deficit. On the basis of this evidence, therefore, it must be concluded that the depth-of-processing interpretation does not yet provide much clarification of the nature of age-related memory difficulties.

Automatic and Effortful Processing

A related framework for memory research makes use of a continuum from automatic memory processes on one end, to effortful memory processes on the other end. This continuum is roughly analogous to the distinction between shallow and deep processing in that the amount of resources or effort required, and the demands on capacity, increase as the processing becomes deeper or more effortful.

Many of the arguments raised with respect to the processing-depth interpretation can also be used in support of this effort interpretation, but as we have seen, the evidence cannot yet be considered very favorable. It has also been argued that recognition tests are less demanding of processing effort and thus might be expected to reveal smaller age differences than recall tests. However, as was pointed out earlier, recognition tests do not always yield equivalent performance across age groups and most recognition-recall comparisons to date have been confounded with task difficulty, and thus this evidence cannot be considered convincing.

Frequency Judgments. One substantive research area in which the processing-effort interpretation has been subjected to direct experimental test is frequency or recency judgments. It has been assumed that registration of the frequency with which an item has occurred is an automatic process requiring little or no cognitive effort, and thus accuracy of frequency or recency judgments should be the same across all age groups. Three studies (Attig & Hasher, 1980; Kausler & Puckett, 1980a; Perlmutter et al., 1981) confirmed this expectation in finding no age differences with a pair-discrimination procedure, but two subsequent studies with the same basic procedure (e.g., Kausler, Hakami, & Wright, 1982; Kausler, Wright & Hakami, 1981) and two studies (e.g., Hasher & Zacks, 1979; Warren & Mitchell, 1980) with a frequency-rating procedure did find age differences in favor of young adults. Until these conflicts are resolved the existing results must be considered only partially consistent with the prediction from the processing-effort interpretation. One can also question whether frequency judgments are truly automatic since a recent study indicated that the accuracy of frequency discrimination was impaired by the performance of a concurrent task, as though both tasks were competing for the same limited capacity and neither was capacity-independent (i.e., Kausler, Wright, & Hakami, 1981).

Other Automatic Memory Processes. Memory for other nonsemantic attributes assumed to be processed automatically, i.e., without cognitive effort, was investigated by Kausler and Puckett (1980b; 1981a; 1981b), McCormack (1981, 1982), Park, Puglisi, and Lutz (1982), Perlmutter et al. (1981), and Waddell and Rogoff (1981). Contrary to prediction, older adults were significantly poorer than young adults in memory for the case (upper or lower) of visually presented words (Kausler & Puckett, 1980b; 1981b), and for the sex of the voice (male or female) of auditorially presented sentences (Kausler & Puckett, 1981a; 1981b). Contradictory results have been reported for memory of spatial location of visually presented items as Park et al. (1982) and Perlmutter et al. (1981) found an advantage for young adults, Waddell and Rogoff (1981) found older adults inferior to middle-aged adults in one task but equivalent in a second task, and young and old adults were equivalent in location accuracy in experiments by McCormack (1982). McCormack (1981) did find comparable performance in young (ages 18–19 years) and old (ages 63–74 years) adults in a measure of the accuracy of temporal location of earlier presented words that appears conceptually similar to the recency-judgment measure employed by earlier investigators.

It has sometimes been argued that the existence of age differences in a memory process indicates that that type of memory is effortful because automatic processes are, by definition, age insensitive. This reasoning is clearly circular, however, and precludes the possibility of ever testing the hypothesis that automatic memory processes are unaffected by adult age. In fairness, it must be pointed out that other criteria, such as a superiority of intentional over incidental learning, were consistent with the conclusion that the case and sex-of-voice attributes do require cognitive effort.

It might well be argued that much of the research discussed earlier under the topics of encoding and semantic memory is consistent with the processing-effort interpretation in that the formation of imaginal mediators or the organization of information requires deep, effortful processing, whereas semantic activation may be automatic. While this may be true, the evidence examined above is equivocal with respect to the automatic-effortful hypothesis as it currently stands, and it is doubtful that subsuming additional results under this interpretation would lead to a greater understanding of the phenomena of interest.

An assessment of the effortful-automatic distinction with respect to memory performance in adulthood must conclude that it has little support at the present time. The evidence with respect to recency or frequency judgments is only moderately consistent within a paradigm (and much less so across paradigms), and several attempts at identifying other automatic processes that are age invariant have not been very successful. Moreover, the distinction is primarily descriptive, and explanations of the cause of age decrements in effortful processes have relied exclusively on vague notions of an age-related reduction in "processing capacity," a concept which has not yet received a satisfactory operational definition (see Chapter 9).

Theoretical Evaluation

A number of researchers have suggested that older adults are less effective in employing mnemonic techniques, and in performance on memory tasks in general, because they are long removed from the type of academic environment that stresses memorizing skills. Following this reasoning, one might expect little or no age differences on measures of "basic" memory, but sizable age differences on measures that stress organizational or mediational strategies. Some support for this expectation is available in the research literature, although the existence of reliable age differences in incidental-learning tasks weakens this argument.

Another implication of the disuse perspective is that individuals who have continuously used their memory abilities should exhibit smaller age declines than those who have not been active memorizers. Murrell and Humphries (1978) reported that this was indeed the case for simultaneous language translators whose job requires that they remember what is said in one language long enough to convert it to speech in another language.

Young (mean age 25 years) and older (mean age 57 years) adults who were either naive or experienced in simultaneous translating were administered a speech-shadowing task. The experienced translators exhibited no age difference in accuracy (22% vs. 23% errors), but the inexperienced older adults were much less accurate than the inexperienced younger adults (59% vs. 35% errors). While quite suggestive, the possibility that the people who have lasted long enough on the job to become experienced were unrepresentative of the general population in terms of initial level of ability should make one cautious about attaching too much significance to this finding.

Perhaps the strongest argument raised in support of a disuse interpretation of memory problems associated with aging is the demonstration that some of the deficits can be overcome by relatively short intervention programs. For example, three recent studies have reported quite dramatic memory improvements with relatively brief training in samples of older adults (Langer, Rodin, Beck, Weinman, & Spitzer, 1979; Schmitt, Murphy, & Sanders, 1981; Zarit, Cole, & Guider, 1981). While encouraging with respect to the modifiability of behavior in later life, these studies are of limited usefulness for determining the causes of age-associated memory problems because only one age group was involved. In order to argue that disuse is a major factor contributing to age differences, it is necessary to demonstrate that older adults improve more than young adults on a measure of memory that does not have a low performance ceiling. Simple repetition or practice is one intervention that has been examined in several age groups, but the currently available evidence suggests that older adults benefit no more from practice on at least some memory tasks than do young adults (Murphy et al., 1981; Taub, 1973; Taub & Long, 1972).

One of the most plausible of the biologically oriented interpretations of age differences in memory is based on the hypothesis that nearly every mental operation requires more time with increased age. Whether this is termed a "slower tempo" (Waugh & Barr, 1980) or a "reduced processing rate" (Salthouse, 1980; Salthouse & Kail, in press), it is obvious that if encoding, organizing, rehearsal, retrieval, etc., take more time in some individuals than in others the resulting memory performance will generally be poorer in the slower individuals. Indeed, Waugh and Barr (1980) have suggested that:

> Dichotomies such as "episodic" versus "semantic" or "primary" versus "secondary" or "deep" versus "superficial" may possibly prove useful in accounting for age-related memory decrements. They will surely not be sufficient. The "slow tempo" principle may even make them unnecessary. (p. 258)

The major limitation of the processing-rate hypothesis of age differences in memory is that at the present time the amount of directly relevant evidence is still rather limited. However, the evidence that does exist appears quite consistent with this perspective. For example, it was noted in the previous chapter that the activation of information in memory requires more time with increasing age. It has also been reported with two independent procedures that the rate of rehearsing information in memory is slower in older adults than in young adults (Salthouse, 1980; Sanders et al., 1980). There are also some reports (e.g., Horn et al., 1981) indicating that measures of rate of processing are moderately correlated with measures of primary and secondary memory, and indices of mnemonic organization.

Two experiments by Nebes (Nebes, 1976; Nebes & Andrews-Kulis, 1976) are sometimes cited as providing evidence against the processing-rate perspective, but a close examination reveals that neither study is particularly convincing. In both studies it was claimed that there were no age differences in the speed of mediator formation, but Nebes (1976) failed to include short enough time intervals to provide a sensitive test of this hypothesis, and Nebes and Andrews-Kulis (1976) actually found older adults to require more than 1 second longer than young adults (i.e., an average of 3.68 vs. 2.60 seconds) to construct integrative sentences relating two words.

An evaluation of memory research with respect to the competence-performance dimension is faced with many of the same problems found to confront the disuse-biological deterioration issue. In order to demonstrate that older adults have the same competence as young adults and are simply performing at a lower level because of less efficient strategies, one must compare the performance of both young and old adults in a situation where strategy variation is eliminated and there are no artifical limits on the range of performance. As reported earlier in the chapter, mixed results have been obtained with attempts to induce imagery, organization, or "deep processing" in adults of different ages and thus it is not yet possible to reach a conclusion concerning the exact nature of the age differences observed in memory functioning.

Perhaps the strongest conclusion that can be drawn concerning the theoretical classification of age differences in memory processes is that a variety of specific mechanisms, rather than a single general mechanism, are likely to be responsible for the observed age effects. The reason is the many different aspects of memory that have been discovered, and the evidence indicates that increased age has different patterns of effects across the various aspects. Correlational evidence should also be relevant to this issue as the presence of high intertask correlations would support a single memory factor, while low correlations would favor multiple, independent memory processes. Unfortunately, the few studies that have reported intertask correlations (e.g., Botwinick & Storandt, 1974a; Kausler & Puckett, 1981b; Perlmutter, 1978; Perlmutter et al., 1981) have typically failed to provide information about the reliabilities (within-task correlations) of the measures and thus the between-task correlations are not easily interpretable. Nevertheless, factor-analytic investigations with adults of varying ages (Botwinick & Storandt, 1974a; Robertson-Tchabo & Arenberg, 1976) have identified at least three distinct memory factors in which paired-associate performance, free-recall performance, and memory-span performance play important roles.

Summary

Two conclusions seem warranted from the research summarized above. One is that no single conceptualization of memory functioning has been markedly successful in isolating the age impairment to a single process or mechanism. Whether the focus has been on interference, stages, stores, processing levels, or automatic versus effortful processing, the research evidence has not been consistent with the specific localization of age differences in only one theoretical process. The reviews of the evidence for various theoretical positions have necessarily been succinct, and undoubtedly proponents of each could provide interpretations of many of the negative findings. The overall impression, however, is that the existing theories have not yet been very useful for precisely localizing the age deficit in memory.

Despite this somewhat negative outcome, these formulations have provided several plausible directions for research. Indeed, the second conclusion, that some aspects of memory functioning appear to be more affected by age than others, is primarily based on research generated from one or the other of the theoretical conceptualizations. Certain aspects, such as the use and efficiency of imaginal mediators and stimulus organization, and processing at "deep" and "effortful" levels to encode in secondary memory, seem to present particular problems for older adults. Other aspects either are unaffected by aging, e.g., intermediate-duration storage between acquisition and test, or cannot be unambiguously evaluated at this time, e.g., retrieval, primary memory, and shallow or automatic processing. This pattern of findings presents a challenge for any proposed explanation since the successful candidate explanation must be able to account not only for the memory aspects that do exhibit age differences, but also for those that do not.

The discovery that sizable age differences are evident with incidental-learning procedures also serves to provide some constraints on the types of explanations that might be proposed. For example, since older adults apparently exhibit performance deficits even when the learning is unintentional, simple monolithic explanations based on motivational or anxiety differences will probably not provide satisfactory interpretations of age-related memory losses.

8. Stimulus Registration and Interpretation

The current chapter deals with selected topics in visual perception. Perception is a very broad term, however, and thus it is desirable to begin with a brief statement as to the type of topics that will, and will not, be considered in the present context. Primarily because of space limitations, only research involving "higher" perceptual processes within the visual modality will be discussed. Restricting one's coverage to visual perception is commonly justified by authors of books in cognition and perception because a disproportionate amount of the research on perceptual processes has focused on vision rather than any of the other sense modalities. This is not quite so true in research on aging as there have been numerous investigations of adult age differences in auditory processes, but it is still the case that the majority of the research of interest to cognitive psychologists has employed visually presented stimuli. Studies primarily concerned with sensory factors will be ignored because the amount of relevant material is so vast that entire books have recently appeared on this topic (e.g., Colavita, 1978; Corso, 1981), and to attempt to do justice to this topic would take us too far from the major focus on cognitive processes.

The material that will be covered in the current chapter can be broadly organized into spatial, temporal, and sensitivity aspects of perception. The former includes topics such as perceptual organization, spatial manipulation, geometrical illusions, and selective attention. Within the temporal category are the topics of motion judgment, temporal fusion and integration, and visual masking. The final section will examine the major results concerning adult age differences in sensitivity to light (detection) and pattern (discrimination).

Spatial Aspects of Perception

Among the most dramatic age differences noted in the discussion of psychometric intelligence in Chapter 4 were those evident in the measures of spatial abilities. On the average, adults in their 60s were found to perform at only about 70%–80% the level of adults in their 20s on the Object Assembly, Picture Arrangement, Picture Completion, and Block Design subtests of the WAIS (see Figures 4.8–4.11). These results have been confirmed in other measurements of spatial ability (see pages 61–64), and thus it is clear that increased age is generally associated with reduced spatial perceptual ability.

A first step in attempting to determine the exact nature of the age-related difficulty in spatial perception is to classify the types of activities required in various tests of spatial ability. One possible classification scheme is based on a distinction among analysis, integration, and manipulation. Analysis operations are required when the individual is expected to locate a specific component within a large configuration, or to identify a missing or unusual component within a scene or complex figure. Integration skills are needed to synthesize complete figures from jumbled or partial segments. And finally, manipulation or transformation abilities are implicated in the performance of tasks involving the comparison of different perspectives of an object or environment.

The present classification scheme is not based on factor analytic investigations, and indeed studies employing sophisticated correlational analyses have generally revealed somewhat different factors (e.g., McGee, 1979). Nevertheless, the current three-factor scheme is useful because the "factors" are intuitively plausible and conceptually distinct, and (most importantly) because the experimental research involving adults of different ages can be easily organized into these three aspects.

Analysis

A variety of results suggest that older adults are poorer at analysis tasks than young adults. The WAIS Picture Completion Test can be considered to require detailed analysis or decomposition of the total pattern in order to identify the missing element, and Figure 4.9 indicates that older adults are generally slower or less accurate than young adults on this test. Other common tests requiring analysis of complex patterns are the Embedded Figures Test and the Gottschaldt Hidden Figures Test in which the individual is required to locate a simple pattern embedded in a more complex pattern. At least nine studies using tests such as these have found older adults to be less accurate, or to require more time, than young adults (e.g., Axelrod & Cohen, 1961; Basowitz & Korchin, 1957; Bogard, 1974; Botwinick & Storandt, 1974a; Chown, 1961; Eisner, 1972; Lee & Pollack, 1978; Panek, Barrett, Sterns, & Alexander, 1978; Schwartz & Karp, 1967).

Another type of test that appears to require a similar type of analytical ability is perception of reversible stimuli. A number of ambiguous figures have been constructed in which two alternative perceptions are possible, and three studies (Botwinick, 1965; Botwinick, Robbin, & Brinley, 1959; Silverman & Reimanis, 1966) have reported that older adults are less likely than young adults to perceive both percepts in the figure. The second percept can be considered analogous to an embedded figure, and thus these results are consistent with those found in more traditional tests of embedded-figure perception.

The situation with respect to ambiguous figure perception is actually not quite this simple as two recent experiments have found no age difference in the *rate* of figure reversals (e.g., Kline, Culler, & Sucec, 1977; Kline, Hogan, & Stier, 1980, Exp. 2), and one experiment actually reported more reversals in older adults than in young adults (i.e., Kline et al. 1980, Exp. 1). The apparent contradiction may be attributable to different processes contributing to the initial reorganization of the figure, and to the rate of subsequent fluctuations between alternative organizations once the first reorganization has been achieved.

There have been a number of speculations offered as to why older adults have difficulty in analyzing parts of complex figures, e.g., they are more distracted by the irrelevant segments or they have problems discriminating figure from ground, but there is not yet any explanation which has received even a moderate amount of empirical support.

Integration

A situation similar to that found with analysis ability exists with respect to tests of the ability to integrate parts into a whole in that there is convincing evidence of age-associated declines with little understanding of the underlying reasons. The WAIS Object Assembly Test requires the individual to assemble a complete object from separate parts in much the same way as a jigsaw puzzle, and Figure 4.8 indicates that older adults are generally poorer at this task than young adults. Other tests requiring integration abilities are the Gestalt Completion Test and the Street Incomplete Figures Test in which individuals are asked to identify pictures that have had various portions deleted. A number of studies have reported an age-related deficiency, either in time or errors, in performance on this type of test (e.g., Basowitz & Korchin, 1957; Crook, Alexander, Anderson, Coules, Hanson, & Jeffries, 1958; Danziger & Salthouse, 1978; Dirken, 1972; Eisner, 1972; Glanzer et al. 1958; Thomas & Charles, 1964; Verville & Cameron, 1946). Only Danziger and Salthouse (1978) attempted to investigate possible causes for these age differences, and their conclusions were mainly negative, i.e., the poorer performance of older adults did not seem attributable to response bias, differential familiarity with the materials, or inefficient distribution of attention across stimulus components.

Kline and his colleagues (e.g., Kline et al., 1977; Kline et al., 1980) have recently examined age differences on a word version of the incomplete figure test, one in which the boundaries of letters are either ill-defined or completely absent. In the first experiment in this series there were three groups of adults with mean ages of 19, 45, and 70 years. The young adults averaged 86% correct identification of the partial words, but the middle-aged and older adults averaged only 14% and 2%, respectively. However, two later experiments (both reported in Kline et al., 1980) found much smaller age differences (i.e., 98% vs. 91%, and 95% vs. 85% for young (ages 18–21) and old (ages 56–87) adults in Experiments 1 and 2, respectively). These later experiments were very similar to the first one except that the words were presented in a slightly different typescript. The format of the letters may therefore be an important factor contributing to the magnitude of the age differences in this particular task. It would now be desirable to conduct a study in which the legibility of the items is systematically manipulated in the same groups of young and old adults to confirm that letter format is, in fact, the major determinant of the age difference in perceiving such inconspicuous stimuli.

One interesting attempt to identify the specific nature of the age difficulty in spatial integration was reported by Ludwig (1982). Stimulus figures composed of six line segments were presented either sequentially or simultaneously in two spatially separated parts. If older adults are hampered at integration or synthesis tasks because of memory problems, one might expect the age differences to be smaller when the two parts are presented at the same time compared to when the parts are presented one after the other. While the reasoning is plausible, Ludwig's results revealed that neither young (mean age 21 years) nor older (mean age 68 years) adults had poorer performance with sequential rather than simultaneous presentation, and thus this particular memory manipulation was evidently not very powerful. Nevertheless analytical investigations of this type will be necessary if one hopes to determine the causes for the dramatic age differences in spatial integration tasks (e.g., 35% vs. 16% correct reproductions for the young and old groups, respectively, in Experiment I of Ludwig's study).

Manipulation

More dynamic aspects of spatial perception are required by tests of perspective taking or mental rotation. Experimental investigations of these abilities are quite recent, but the available studies are fairly consistent in indicating age-associated deficits in both activities. For example, one experiment (Herman & Coyne, 1980) found young (mean age 24 years) adults to be superior to old (mean ages 65 and 75 years) adults in the accuracy of localizing objects from imagined perspectives. A series of three experiments by Ohta, Walsh, and Krauss (1981) also investigated spatial perspective-taking skills in adults of varying ages, and found older adults to be generally less accurate and to require more time than young adults. These investigators attempted to identify the nature of the age difficulty by examining performance across different classes of inappropriate perspectives, but a significant age by incorrect alternative interaction was found in only one of six comparisons (i.e., two dependent measures in each of three experiments). Therefore, the major conclusion warranted from the Ohta et al. (1981) study simply seems to be that older adults have greater difficulty, for still unspecified reasons, than young adults at imagining different perspectives.

Shepard (e.g., Shepard & Metzler, 1971) introduced a paradigm for investigating the rate of mental rotation that has been employed in four studies with adults of varying ages. Gaylord and Marsh (1976) used the same stimuli (i.e., pairs of line drawings of three-dimensional figures in different perspectives), and task [i.e., classification of the pairs as "same" (identical figures) or "different" (mirror image figures) as rapidly as possible], as Shepard and Metzler (1971). The function relating classification time to degree of angular discrepancy between the stimulus pairs has been found to be quite linear, and thus the rate of mental rotation can be inferred from the slope of this function. The primary result from the Gaylord and Marsh (1976) study was that older (ages 65–72 years) adults had slower rates of rotation than young (ages 18–24 years) adults (i.e., 17.7 msec/degree vs. 8.1 msec/degree). A subsequent experiment by Jacewicz and Hartley (1979) failed to confirm the slope difference with slightly different procedures, but their older adults were only 52–62 years of age. That this was probably an important difference is suggested by a recent extension of the Jacewicz and Hartley study with a more senior (i.e., mean age 72 years) group of older adults in which the original Gaylord and Marsh result of slower rates of mental rotation with increased age was confirmed (Cerella, Poon, & Fozard, 1981). Berg, Hertzog, and Hunt (1982) also reported that the mental rotation rate increased monotonically across age groups with mean ages of 21, 32, 51, and 63 years. This latter finding is particularly convincing since the same trend was evident across four sessions of practice involving 480 trials each.

Selective Attention

Another potentially important aspect of spatial perception concerns the ability to focus selectively on certain stimulus features while ignoring other, irrelevant features. One of the most widely cited studies in the psychology of aging literature is an experiment on selective-attention ability by Rabbitt (1965a). A card-sorting task was used in which young (mean age 19 years) and old (mean age 67 years) adults were requested to sort cards into two piles on the basis of whether an A or a B was present on the card. In different conditions either 0, 1, 4, or 8 irrelevant letters were also present in various locations on the card. It was reported that an increase in the number of irrelevant items led to a greater absolute increase in card-sorting time among older adults (i.e., from .63 to 1.16 sec/card with 0 to 8 irrelevant items) than young adults (i.e., from .38 to .65 sec/card).

However, the exact interpretation of the Rabbitt (1965a) result is not yet clear. It is commonly found that the absolute age difference in time increases with increased task difficulty, apparently regardless of the specific manipulation employed to influence difficulty (cf. Salthouse, in press), and thus one cannot simply attribute this finding to an age-related difficulty in ignoring irrelevant items. Furthermore, relative rather than absolute measures of performance did not increase systematically with an increase in the number of irrelevant items. That is, the ratio of card-sorting time of older adults to card-sorting time of young adults was 1.66 for 0 irrelevant items, 1.25 for 1 irrelevant item, 1.56 for 4 irrelevant items, and 1.78 for 8 irrelevant items. No statistical evaluation of these ratios is available but this method of analysis, which may be more meaningful than the comparison of absolute performance times, is not consistent with the hypothesis that older adults are more affected by increased number of irrelevant items than young adults.

A similar problem is evident in a more recent elaboration of Rabbitt's (1965a) experiment by Farkas and Hoyer (1980). These investigators compared the effects of irrelevant items that varied in the similarity of orientation to the relevant items and found that older adults had greater absolute increases in card-sorting time than younger adults with each manipulation. However, once again ratio comparisons were not statistically evaluated, and the data in the figures presented in the report appear to indicate roughly constant old/young ratios across conditions.

An experiment by Wright and Elias (1979) raised the question of whether there is an age difference in the ability to ignore, rather than merely discriminate, irrelevant items by eliminating the positional uncertainty of the target. Target letters were presented in the middle of the visual field, and in different conditions the target was either alone or flanked by neutral letters, by letters designating the same response, or by letters designating the opposite response. The various manipulations were effective in altering reaction time, but comparable effects of the presence of irrelevant letters were found in young (age 18–25 years) and old (age 60–82 years) adults. The authors concluded that there may be an age deficit in competition between alternative responses, but that both young and old adults are equally able to ignore irrelevant features of a stimulus array.

It is unfortunate that there is not less ambiguous evidence concerning age differences in selective attention as this ability might be a major factor in tests of analysis and integration. However, at the present time no definite conclusion can be reached concerning the effects of adult age on the focusing on specific elements in the spatial environment. There is still some question about whether absolute, rather than relative, age comparisons are adequate for making interpretations of age differences, and a study eliminating discrimination processes in selective attention revealed no age differences.

Miscellaneous

Several other aspects of spatial perception have also been investigated in adults of varying ages, but the results from such studies have not yet been impressive enough to warrant firm conclusions. For example, three studies have reported contradictory results on the effect of body position on judgments of rod verticality in adults of different ages. Comalli, Wapner, and Werner (1959) and Girotti and Beretta (1969) found young adults to shift the apparent vertical to the opposite direction of one's body tilt, while older adults judged a rod to be vertical when it was aligned in the same direction as the body orientation. However, Davies and Laytham (1964) reported that adults in all age groups from 20–79 years located the vertical in the side opposite of the body tilt. It is not clear why these studies would yield different results, although the subjective nature of the judgment is probably responsible for some of the variability.

A report by Brebner (1962) indicated that older adults (mean age 74 years) were less accurate than young adults (mean age 21 years) in absolute judgments of line length, but a later experiment with a magnitude estimation procedure revealed no age differences in line estimations (Verillo, 1981). Moreover, Miles (1935) reported age invariance in his analyses of spatial estimation data originally collected by Galton. Correlations involving over 3000 adults between the ages of 25 and 81 years were: age and perpendicularity error = .06; age and bisection error = .07; and age and trisection error = .03. It thus appears that there are no pronounced age differences in these two-dimensional aspects of space perception, although there is some evidence that depth perception may be slightly impaired with increased age (e.g., Bell, Wolf, & Berholz, 1972; Jani, 1966).

Another area of spatial perception that has been the focus of considerable research is susceptibility to various geometrical illusions. Unfortunately this area has also contributed little to the understanding of age differences in perception; in this case because the results have been rather inconsistent, and because no well-accepted explanations of the factors responsible for the various illusions are yet available. The most research has been done with the Mueller-Lyer (double arrow) Illusion, with several studies reporting increased illusion with increased age (e.g., Atkeson, 1978; Frederickson & Geurin, 1973; Wapner, Werner, & Comalli, 1960), but others reporting unsystematic age effects (e.g., Barclay & Comalli, 1970; Eisner, 1972). Wapner, Werner, and Comalli (1960) reported smaller Titchener (satellite circles) Illusion magnitude in older adulthood, but two later studies (e.g., Coren & Porac, 1978; Eisner, 1972) found insignificant age trends. The Delboef (concentric circles) Illusion was reported to yield comparable illusion effects between the ages of 21 and 46 (Sjostrom & Pollack, 1971), but both to decrease (Lorden, Atkeson, & Pollack, 1979) and increase (Pollack & Atkeson, 1978) with increased age between the ages of 25 and 75 years. A trend of stability until middle age followed by reduced susceptibility in older age has been reported for the Ponzo (converging lines) Illusion (e.g., Farquhar & Leibowitz, 1971; Leibowitz & Judisch, 1967).

Substantial age-related impairments in spatial aspects of perception have been consistently reported whenever there is a requirement for some type of active cognitive processing. The processing can be analysis, integration, or manipulation, but in each case performance seems to be adversely affected by increased age. It is not yet clear whether perceptual activities that may involve lesser amounts of processing, such as some forms of selective attention and judgments of lines, angles, and geometrical illusions, are also affected by increasing age.

Temporal Aspects of Perception

Many stimuli are limited in the duration that they are available in the environment and thus visual perception can be as dependent upon the temporal, as upon the spatial, dimension. This is particularly true when the relevant stimulus is in motion, but it is also the case when a stationary stimulus is only available briefly because of rapidly changing environmental conditions or motion on the part of the observer. In this section we will examine the evidence relevant to adult age differences in these processes.

Motion Judgment

Perhaps the temporal task with the most obvious practical relevance involves anticipating the future position of a moving object. Crook, Devoe, Hageman, Hanson, Krulee, and Ronco (1957) first investigated age differences in this ability in the context of judgments about the possible collision of simulated airplanes. This was a very careful study involving 165 healthy males between the ages of 15 and 59 years of age, none of whom had had prior flying experience. With increased age more time was needed to make the decision concerning whether or not the approaching aircraft were on a collision course. Approximately 1 additional second was required by the 50-year-olds compared to the 20-year-olds, which the authors claim would be equivalent to about 1/3 of a mile closer to collision if the two aircraft had speeds of 600 miles per hour. This reduced safety margin would obviously have important consequences if comparable results were to be found with experienced pilots.

Hills (1980) has reported a similar age-related deficit in motion judgments concerning automobiles. Older adults (ages 61–70 years) were found to be less sensitive than young adults (ages 31–40 years) at estimating the speed of approaching vehicles at an intersection.

Two studies employing artificial laboratory tasks have also been consistent in demonstrating poorer position anticipation with increased age. One of these (Haywood, 1980) compared a group of young adults (mean age 23 years) with two groups of older adults (means ages 68 and 72 years) in the accuracy of pressing a button when an object, simulated by sequentially illuminated lamps, reached a predesignated position. The young adults averaged .049 second absolute anticipation error, whereas the two groups of older adults had average errors of .075 and .089 seconds. A similar finding of greater errors in older adults (mean age 69 years) than in young adults (mean age 23 years) was reported by Salthouse and Somberg (1982c) in a task designed to resemble an activity from a video game. A target crossed a display screen on a horizontal trajectory, and the individual attempted to initiate a projectile on a vertical trajectory such that the two trajectories would intersect one another at the same point in time (i.e., the target was shot down). The older adults scored fewer hits than the young adults, and there was no trend for this age difference to become smaller across 600 trials of experience.

Although there is remarkable consensus concerning the existence of age differences in the accuracy of judgments about moving objects, there is still very little known about the reasons for these differences. It seems unlikely that the older adults were limited by basic sensory processes since the stimuli were well above threshold and were displayed for a period of at least 1 second. (However in a later section we will learn that older adults have poorer acuity for moving objects even when they are equivalent to young adults on static acuity.) There is some evidence (e.g., Shagass, Amadeo, & Overton, 1974; Sharpe & Sylvester, 1978) that the eye movements of older adults lag behind moving stimuli to a greater extent than those of young adults, and the inability to maintain continuous visual contact with the moving stimulus may be contributing to the poorer performance of older adults. Another possibility, consistent with results in a variety of other tasks, is that the mental computation of the projected trajectory requires more time with increased age such that older adults were less likely to correctly complete the mental computations by the time the relevant action was required.

Tachistoscopic Perception

Some of the most dramatic age differences reported in cognitive psychology tasks are found in the accuracy of identifying briefly presented stimuli. The poorer performance of older adults was first described by Miles (1933), and the basic result has been confirmed in many subsequent studies with a great variety of stimuli (e.g., Charman, 1979; Eriksen, Hamlin, & Breitmeyer, 1970; Eriksen & Steffy, 1964; Rajalakshmi & Jeeves, 1963; Wallace, 1956). This phenomenon of age-related increases in the duration required to perceive a single (unmasked) stimulus has also been frequently reported in most (e.g., Coyne, 1981; Kline & Birren, 1975; Kline & Szafran, 1975; Till, 1978; Walsh, 1976; Walsh, Till, & Williams, 1978) but not all (e.g., Hertzog, Williams, & Walsh, 1976; Till & Franklin, 1981; Walsh, Williams, & Hertzog, 1979) visual masking studies.

Many of the recent investigations of age differences in tachistoscopic perception have utilized a procedure involving the successive presentation of two or more short-duration stimuli. Figure 8.1 illustrates the basic paradigm and the two major mechanisms that appear to be responsible for performance

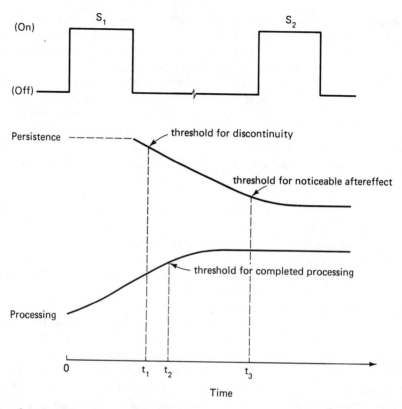

Figure 8.1. Proposed model for persistence and processing mechanisms in successive stimulation conditions. S1 and S2 refer to two successively presented visual stimuli. Time increases from left to right in all panels.

in such multiple-stimulus tasks. The top portion of the figure illustrates the temporal sequencing of the two stimuli. The interval between S1 and S2 is usually manipulated as an independent variable or measured as a dependent variable. The middle panel of Figure 8.1 represents the neural residual of the physical stimulus, sometimes referred to as iconic memory. Formation of an internal representation, or the process of stimulus encoding, is portrayed in the bottom panel of Figure 8.1.

It is important to note that Figure 8.1 incorporates several specific assumptions that may eventually be proved inaccurate. For example, persistence is represented as beginning at the point of stimulus offset, and yet there is some evidence (e.g., DiLollo, 1980) that it may actually begin at stimulus onset. Also, the efficiency of processing is assumed to be independent of the quantity or quality of information in the persistence, but it is possible that processing efficiency is directly related to the level of persistence. And finally, the relationships illustrated in Figure 8.1 suggest that the persistence provides the raw material for processing, at least after the offset of the stimulus. An alternative possibility is that rather than serving as the basis for processing, the persistence is itself a product or consequence of some form of processing.

Although these particular details may eventually have to be altered, Figure 8.1 is useful for clarifying the relationships among several different experimental tasks. Tasks requiring identification of single stimuli can be conceived of as involving a race between rate of processing and decay of persistence, whereas judgments concerning the perceived duration of stimuli would be primarily dependent upon the time course of the persistence mechanism.

Moreover, following Hawkins and Shulman (1979), two different types of persistence judgments can be distinguished. One type has to do with the detection of a noticeable difference from the physical stimulus, or the perception of discontinuity in two or more discrete stimuli. The second type of persistence judgment is based on the point at which the sensory residual is no longer detectable, or distinguishable from no persistence. In a sense, the former judgment concerns the perceived duration of the external stimulus, while the latter relates to the duration of the stimulus aftereffect within the nervous system. This distinction is primarily qualitative, in that the two types of persistence judgments are assumed to involve different kinds of information. However, quantitative variations are also possible within each type of judgment as the exact location of the threshold region would be expected to vary with a multitude of sensory and decision factors.

Critical Fusion Frequency. The rate of alternation between light and dark that just leads to the transition between flicker and fusion is known as the critical fusion frequency (CFF). In terms of Figure 8.1, the critical fusion frequency is probably equivalent to the threshold for discontinuity. This type of judgment can apparently be made quite easily, as the reliability coefficients are often reported to be above .9 (e.g., Misiak, 1951; Wilson, 1963). A large number of factors have been found to influence the critical fusion frequency (e.g., size, brightness and retinal locus of the target, ratio of light to dark in the flicker cycle, state of dark adaptation, and presence or absence of an artifical pupil), but most values for young adults are in the range of 30 to 50 cycles per second. Since the most frequent cycle ratio is 50% light and 50% dark, these values correspond to dark intervals between successive light flashes of approximately 10 to 17 msec (i.e., 50 cycles per second is equivalent to one cycle in 20 msec, and 50% of 20 msec is 10 msec).

It is now well-established that increased age is associated with a reduction in the critical fusion frequency, i.e., an increase in the dark interval between light flashes while still perceiving a continuous light. Figure 8.2 illustrates the results from studies including three or more age groups with adults ranging from 20 to 75 years. Additional experiments indicating fewer cycles per second in order to perceive continuity among older adults relative to young adults were reported by Botwinick and Brinley (1963), Falk and Kline (1978),

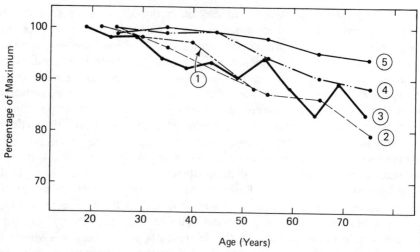

Figure 8.2. Critical fusion frequency at various ages expressed as a percentage of the maximum across all ages. Numbers refer to different experiments: 1 = adapted from Brozek & Keys (1945); 2 = adapted from Coppinger (1955); 3 = adapted from Misiak (1951); 4 = adapted from McFarland, Warren, & Karis (1958); and 5 = adapted from Wilson (1963).

Huntington and Simonson (1965), Misiak (1947), Simonson, Anderson, and Keiper (1967), and Simonson, Enzer, and Blankstein (1941). A notable exception to this declining trend was reported by Szafran (1968) who found a correlation of only −.04 between age and critical fusion frequency for 189 healthy male pilots between the ages of 20 and 60. No reason is yet available for this discrepant result.

A two-stimulus version of the critical fusion procedure involving a discrimination between one and two light flashes was investigated by Amberson, Atkeson, Pollack, and Malatesta (1979) and DiLollo, Arnett, and Kruk (1982). Older adults relative to young adults were again found to require more time between flashes before they could perceive two distinct stimuli, but for some unknown reason the thresholds for this task were on the order of 50–70 msec rather than the 10–17 msec typically reported with the multiple-stimulus version of the critical fusion frequency task. Nevertheless, it is clear that increased age is accompanied by a greater refractoriness to successive stimulation, and that as a consequence older adults are less able to distinguish between temporally discrete events than are young adults.

Temporal Integration. The situation is somewhat more equivocal with respect to age differences in the second type of persistence judgment. Our discussion will be restricted to situations in which the stimuli were exposed tachistoscopically for relatively brief durations, although there have been a number of studies, with mixed results, examining age differences in the duration of aftereffects to visual displays of prolonged duration. (For example, Coyne,

Eiler, Vanderplas, and Botwinick, 1979, and Heron and Chown, 1967, found no age differences in aftereffect duration, but Griew, Fellows, and Howes, 1963, and Kline and Nestor, 1977, found greater persistence in older adults.)

Two basic tasks have been employed; one involving different stimuli as S1 and S2, and the other involving the same stimulus for both S1 and S2. When the first and second stimuli are different the task is to attempt to integrate the two stimuli to form a composite stimulus that is then to be identified. The ease of integration is presumed to be dependent upon the quality of information still available in the persistence from the first stimulus at the time of presentation of the second stimulus. In terms of the scheme of Figure 8.1, this task probably involves persistence judgments of the maximal duration of the stimulus aftereffect rather than the initial perception of discontinuity.

The first aging study of this type was an experiment by Kline and Baffa (1976) in which the S1 and S2 stimuli consisted of patterns of dots, each forming a random half of a three-letter word. Accuracy of composite stimulus identification was determined at six interstimulus intervals ranging from 0 to 150 msec. A fairly rigorous screening procedure, employed to ensure that all participants could perceive the composite stimuli in a single presentation, resulted in the elimination of 13 older adults and 4 young adults. The remaining sample of 12 young (mean age 21 years) and 12 old (mean age 56 years) adults were then presented the two stimuli at durations determined by their individual thresholds (i.e., an average of 15 msec for the old, 7 msec for the young). Despite the longer presentation times for the older adults and the select nature of the sample, the older adults were significantly less accurate than the young adults at identifying the composite stimulus at each interstimulus interval.

A later study by Kline and Orme-Rogers (1978) employed stimuli constructed out of line segments rather than dot patterns, and found exactly the opposite result as Kline and Baffa (1976). The highest accuracy was achieved by adults with a mean age of 68 years rather than adults with a mean age of 19 years. No individuals were excluded for failure to recognize composite stimuli in the 1978 experiment, and all participants had perfect identification when the two stimulus components were presented with a 0 msec interstimulus interval. The nature of the stimuli is probably a critical factor in the discrepancy between the studies as the dot pattern stimuli apparently required spatial integration or closure which, as noted earlier, is especially difficult for older adults. However, without results from a single experiment systematically manipulating the nature of the stimuli this interpretation must merely be considered speculation at the present time.

Two experiments employing the same stimulus (S1 = S2) version of the persistence task have also yielded contradictory results. Walsh and Thompson (1978) examined the interstimulus interval at which individuals reported the stimulus (a circle) to be continuously present. The instructions are similar to those in the critical fusion frequency task, but the participants apparently interpreted them to mean that the judgment should concern the longest interval at which some residual of the first stimulus is still detectable because the durations were over 10 times greater than those typically reported in critical fusion frequency tasks.

The major result from the Walsh and Thompson (1978) experiment was that older adults (mean age 67 years) reported shorter persistence than young adults (mean age 24 years) across several conditions of monoptic (same eye) and dichoptic (alternate eyes) exposure and varying stimulus durations (i.e., 10, 50, and 90 msec). On the average, the older adults reported a persistence of 248 msec compared to the 289 msec value reported by the young adults.

The contradictory study was reported by Kline and Schieber (1981a) who followed very similar procedures and yet found older adults (mean age 69 years) to have longer persistence judgments than young adults (mean age 19 years). The reason for this discrepancy is not yet clear, but it is noteworthy that the various studies have not been very consistent in the estimates derived from roughly comparable samples of young adults. For example, in the two conditions of the Kline and Schieber experiment the young adults averaged 183 and 206 msec persistence. The average in the Walsh and Thompson (1978) study was 289 msec, and the young adults in the original study by Haber and Standing (1969) upon which the later experiments were based averaged 386 msec. It is likely that some of the variability in these results is due to the ambiguous instructions and the subjective nature of the data. However, regardless of the exact reasons for the inconsistency, the existing results are inadequate as a basis for a conclusion about adult age differences in iconic persistence.

Visual Masking. Visual masking tasks typically involve the presentation of two successive stimuli with the individual required either to identify the first (backward masking), or the second (forward masking), stimulus. The primary dependent variable is usually the interstimulus interval that is necessary for a given level of accuracy, although the level of accuracy at a fixed interstimulus interval can also be used as a performance index. Since the requirement is to identify one of the two stimuli, performance in visual masking tasks will be dependent upon both the persistence and processing mechanisms illustrated in Figure 8.1.

Forward masking is primarily determined by the persistence mechanism as the likelihood of identification of S2 will vary inversely with the level of persistence remaining from S1. The rate of processing S2 may also influence performance, but it is unlikely that the processing mechanism for the second stimulus can begin until the persistence from the first stimulus has reached some minimum level. Only one experiment has been published comparing adults of different ages in forward masking, but the results of that study appear unambiguous. Coyne (1981) examined the interstimulus interval necessary to achieve four successive identifications of the second stimulus in 24 adults from each of three age groups (mean ages of 25, 64 and 74 years). The average intervals were 25, 52, and 70 msec, respectively, for the three age groups, clearly suggesting that with increased age more time is needed to escape from the residual persistence of the preceding stimulus.

Many more studies have been reported with the backward masking task because it is assumed to provide an estimate of the time necessary to complete the processing of the initial stimulus. Variations in the time of occurrence of S2 should lead to systematic changes in the probability of correct S1 identification, and thus the time course of the processing mechanism can be inferred from backward masking data. Without exception studies comparing backward masking susceptibility in different age groups have found older adults either to be less accurate at a fixed interstimulus interval, or to require a longer interstimulus interval to achieve a fixed level of accuracy, than young adults (e.g., Cerella, Poon, & Fozard, 1982; DiLollo et al., 1982; Kline & Birren, 1975; Kline & Szafran, 1975; Till & Franklin, 1981; Welsandt, Zupnick, & Meyer, 1973).

The results from backward masking experiments in which the data were presented in tabular form are illustrated in Figure 8.3. The data from these separate studies are considered together because the experiments were all very similar in terms of sample characteristics, experimental procedures, tasks, and dependent measures. The axes represent a measure of the S1-S2 interval (i.e., stimulus onset asynchrony or interstimulus interval) necessary to achieve a specified level of accuracy. Two important features should be noted from this figure. The first is simply that all of the data points fall above the positive diagonal, indicating that the older adults always required more time than the young adults. The second, and more intriguing, aspect of Figure 8.3 is that the data suggest that the absolute difference between the times of young and old adults increases monotonically with the time required by the young adults. This is evident in the linear regression slope of 1.85 when the data from all studies are combined. Such a trend was probably not obvious in any single study because each involved only a restricted range of times, and there was considerable variability in the interval estimates because of small sample sizes.

One implication of the trend apparent in Figure 8.3 is that the specific conditions leading to backward masking may be less important as a determinant of the absolute magnitude of the age difference than the overall difficulty of the task, as reflected in the time required by the young adults. For example, one of the major theoretical issues in this area has been whether age differences were comparable in both "peripheral" and "central" masking. (The terms are primarily labels referring to operationally distinct forms of backward masking; there has not yet been any evidence establishing that they have different anatomical loci.) It has been claimed (e.g., Till & Franklin, 1981) that the age differences are greater in central compared to peripheral masking, but this may simply be an artifact of the central masking tasks generally resulting in longer interstimulus intervals than peripheral masking tasks. Indeed, the two studies in Figure 8.3 with the shortest time requirements for young adults, and also the smallest absolute age differences (i.e., Till, 1978; Walsh et al., 1978) involved peripheral masking, while the other three

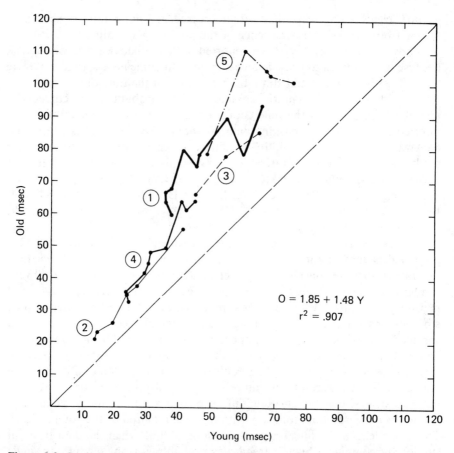

Figure 8.3. Backward masking effectiveness in older adults as a function of backward masking effectiveness in young adults. Each point represents a different condition in the designated report. Numbers refer to different articles: 1 = adapted from Hertzog, Williams, & Walsh (1976); 2 = adapted from Till (1978); 3 = adapted from Walsh (1976); 4 = adapted from Walsh, Till, & Williams (1978); and 5 = adapted from Walsh, Williams, & Hertzog (1979).

studies all involved central masking. The data reported by Till and Franklin are also consistent with this trend (e.g., their Figure 3), as the time requirements and absolute age differences in the central masking task were much greater than those for the peripheral masking task.

A second implication of the trend portrayed in Figure 8.3 is that if age differences increase with increased task complexity, then it is likely that many higher cognitive processes will also be affected by the slower rate of processing associated with increased age. In other words, the more complex the cognitive activity, the greater the likelihood that processing rate will be an important factor contributing to the performance differences between age groups. This inference has also been reached on the basis of similar age trends observed in perceptual-motor tasks (Salthouse, in press).

A reasonable conclusion from the research on visual masking is that the rate of processing visual stimuli is slower with increased age. One would therefore expect age differences to be more pronounced the greater the processing requirements of the task. In fact, there is reasonable support for this prediction at the present time. For example, older adults have been found to suffer more than young adults with increases in the number of items in the display (e.g., Cerella, Poon, & Fozard, 1982; Schonfield & Wenger, 1975; Walsh & Prasse, 1980), and with the requirement to search the array in order to report only items from a specified region of the display (e.g., Salthouse, 1976; Walsh & Thompson, cited in Walsh, 1975). It has also been reported that very large age differences are evident when there is spatial uncertainty as to the location of the target stimulus and some type of visual search process is necessary (e.g., Eriksen & Steffy, 1964; Salthouse & Somberg, 1982c; Somberg & Salthouse, in press; Walsh, Vletas, & Thompson, cited in Walsh & Prasse, 1980).

Age differences appear to be evident in both of the mechanisms portrayed in Figure 8.1. The persistence mechanism is implicated in the age differences in the critical fusion frequency and forward masking tasks, even though there are mixed results concerning other measures of visual persistence. The processing mechanism is assumed to be slower because older adults require more time between successive stimuli in order to identify the first one in the sequence.

Visual Sensitivity

Although the primary focus in this chapter has been on higher perceptual processes, it is important to examine some of the more elementary aspects of perception in order to appreciate the role of peripheral mechanisms in age differences in cognitive processes. The two aspects that will be considered here are detection, the registration of the presence of a stimulus, and discrimination, the identification or resolution of spatial patterns.

Static Acuity

The best known measure of visual sensitivity is acuity or spatial resolving power. This is essentially the ability to discriminate fine details of a spatial pattern as is needed to identify a letter in the Snellen eye chart, or to determine the orientation of the gap in a Landolt C. Although optical corrections can usually improve static acuity, age differences have been noted in both uncorrected and corrected acuity.

Galton (1885) was one of the first to collect systematic data on adult age differences in uncorrected visual acuity, although his results were not published until 1927 by Ruger and Stoessiger. Miles (1935) analyzed these data from 3,250 males between the ages of 25 and 81 years, and reported that the correlation between age and acuity (distance at which type could be read) was −.51. More recently Heron and Chown (1967) examined acuity with the Landolt C procedure at a viewing distance of 6 meters. They found that between the range of 20–79 years, age and uncorrected acuity were correlated −.42 for 300 males, and −.44 for 240 females. These negative values clearly indicate that the ability to resolve spatial detail decreases with increased age.

It is somewhat surprising that corrected vision also exhibits age declines in large population surveys. For example, Chapanis (1950) reported poorer static acuity with increased age in a sample of 574 individuals tested with glasses if they were normally worn. Burg (1966) also found a negative relationship between corrected binocular acuity and age in a sample of 17,500 adults between the ages of 16 and 92 years. The results for the males in this sample

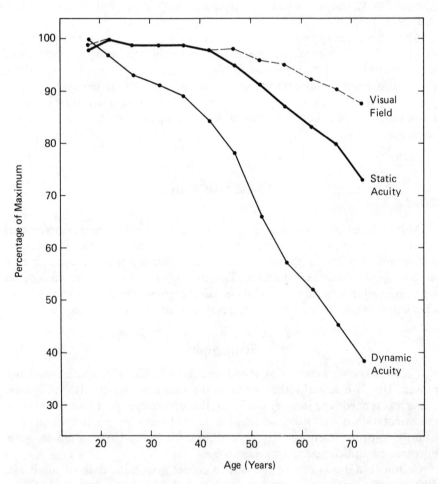

Figure 8.4. Visual sensitivity at various ages expressed as a percentage of the maximum across all ages. Data from Burg (1966, 1968).

are illustrated in Figure 8.4. Notice that there is a slight progressive decrease in visual acuity beginning in the decade of the 40s. It is likely that at least some of this acuity impairment could be eliminated with more frequent prescription changes.

Light Sensitivity

The simplest measure of visual detection is the absolute threshold for determining the presence of light. This clearly varies with the state of dark adaptation and consequently experiments investigating absolute thresholds have typically also reported data on the transition from the unadapted to the completely dark-adapted state. The universal finding in many such studies is that older adults relative to young adults need more light to detect a target at the beginning of adaptation, and that they need even more light after 20–40 minutes of adaptation. Correlations between chronological age and final level of light sensitivity have been reported as high as −.895 (for a sample of 194 males between the ages of 20 and 60—McFarland & Fisher, 1955), with others generally between −.16 (for a sample of 197 male pilots aged 20–60 years— Szafran, 1968) and −.84 (for a sample of 240 males aged 16–89 years— McFarland, Domey, Warren, & Ward, 1960). McFarland and Fisher (1955) have estimated that the amount of light in the target must be doubled for every 13 years of age in order to be just detected by the dark-adapted eye. The basic phenomenon is robust as well as powerful as a number of other studies have reported very similar results with slightly different procedures (e.g., Birren, Bick, & Fox, 1948; Robertson & Yudkin, 1944; Steven, 1946).

The absolute level of light, and the degree of contrast between target and background, are also important in discrimination tasks. Moreover, a number of studies have indicated that variations in light and contrast have greater effects in samples of older adults than in young adults (e.g., Blackwell & Blackwell, 1971; Fortuin, 1963; Guth, 1957; Richards, 1977; Weston, 1948). On the average, adults in their 60s appear to require from two to three times as much total light energy, or as much contrast between targets and background, in order to achieve visual performance comparable to adults in their 20s.

There are also sizable age differences in the disrupting effects of a sudden light producing a glare (e.g., Burg, 1967; Wolf, 1960). This would be expected on the basis of the results just discussed because a light flash reduces the contrast between target and background, and changes the individual's state of dark adaptation such that a recovery time is needed to achieve the prior state of sensitivity.

Many of these differences in basic detection and discrimination are probably attributable to a variety of physical changes that take place in the visual system as one grows older. For example, the loss of lens elasticity reduces the ability to focus on objects at different distances (presbyopia), and this undoubtedly contributes to the poorer uncorrected static acuity. A reduction

in average pupil size (senile miosis), altered spectral transmission characteristics of the lens, and increased opacity of the ocular media all serve to
attenuate the amount of light reaching the retina in older age and thus these
factors are involved in the reduced sensitivity to light. It is not yet known
whether there are actual structural changes in the retina associated with
normal aging.

Visual Field

Another visual change that has been noted to occur with increased age is
a slight shrinkage of the effective field of vision. The average young adult has
a horizontal field of approximately 175 degrees of visual angle, but several
studies indicate that there is a loss of about two degrees per decade beginning
at around age 45 (e.g., Bell, 1972; Ferree, Rand, & Monroe, 1930; Wolf, 1967).
Data from Burg's (1968) large-scale study are illustrated in Figure 8.4. It has
been hypothesized that changes in the prominence of the nose and the relative
location of the eyeball contribute to this loss of peripheral sensitivity, but
confirmatory measurements have apparently not been performed.

Dynamic Visual Acuity

Although the conventional method of measuring acuity involves a stationary observer and a stationary target, acuity can also be measured when there
is relative motion between the observer and the target. As one might expect,
static and dynamic visual acuity are closely related with slow target speeds,
but the correlations drop to about .3 or less with target velocities in excess of
100 degrees/second. Older adults have been found to exhibit more pronounced
acuity drops than young adults with moving targets in at least three experiments (e.g., Farrimond, 1967; Heron & Chown, 1967; Reading, 1972). Burg
(1966) also included measures of dynamic acuity in his survey of California
automobile drivers, and his results for a target velocity of 120 degrees/second
are illustrated in Figure 8.4.

Two more recent studies have also reported special difficulties with moving
targets in older age groups. Sekuler, Hutman, and Owsley (1980) found older
observers (mean age 75 years) to be less sensitive to moving gratings than
young observers (mean age 20 years), despite the two groups having nearly
equivalent static acuity. Sivak, Olson, and Pastalan (1981) also matched
young (ages 18–24 years) and old (ages 62–74 years) adults on high-luminance
static acuity, and then compared them on low-luminance dynamic acuity (i.e.,
ability to distinguish the orientation of the letter E on a highway sign while
riding in an automobile at night). The distance at which the sign was legible
was significantly shorter for the older adults, indicating that the combination
of low luminance and relative motion presented problems above and beyond
those associated with typical static acuity.

Miscellaneous

Sekuler and Hutman (1980) have reported another visual phenomenon that does not appear to be interpretable in terms of simple acuity or light sensitivity factors. These investigators presented observers with bar gratings of different widths to determine the minimum contrast necessary for detection. Young (mean age 19 years) and old (mean age 73 years) participants did not differ in standard clinical acuity tests, and were also found to be equivalent in contrast sensitivity to high spatial frequency (narrow bar) gratings. However, the contrast sensitivity to low spatial frequency (wide bar) gratings was much poorer for the older adults than for the younger ones. This rather counterintuitive finding deserves further attention by researchers as it may prove useful in isolating the neural, rather than simply optical, changes associated with visual aging.

It is indisputable that fundamental biological changes are responsible for most if not all of the age differences reported in visual sensitivity. The association with age is so strong in the case of two of these changes that they have even been labeled with age-specific terms, i.e., senile miosis and presbyopia. What is not yet clear is whether there are also neural changes at the level of the retina or beyond. The findings that older adults are poorer at dynamic visual acuity and low spatial frequency detection even when equivalent to young adults in static acuity suggest that there may be age differences at higher levels in the visual system, but there is apparently no direct physiological or anatomical confirmation of these speculations available at the present time.

Theoretical Evaluation

There is very little basis for making firm theoretical distinctions from the research available in visual perception and aging, but the implicit assumptions of most researchers are that the age differences are maturational in nature, that they are not mere performance factors but instead are reflections of true competence, and that there are several specific mechanisms involved rather than a single general cause. It is possible that a particular type of environmental exposure exacerbates what are normally rather slight age differences, as has been found in the case of age-related loss of auditory sensitivity to high-frequency tones (presbycusis), but the evidence documenting such an effect in the visual modality is not yet available.

The age differences that have been observed in visual perception are presumed to indicate levels of competence because people are highly motivated to maintain their visual abilities. The laboratory tasks assessing spatial and temporal aspects of perception are probably unfamiliar to most people, but no explanations have been offered to account for how unfamiliarity per se could lead to the age differences that have been reported. Because of the variety of perceptual processes that have been found to exhibit age differences (e.g., light sensitivity, dynamic acuity, visual persistence, rate of processing, spatial analysis, spatial integration, etc.), it is assumed that a number of different mechanisms are involved. For example, in addition to peripheral optical factors, several theorists have hypothesized that a stimulus persistence (e.g., Kline & Schieber, 1981b; Pollack, 1978) or visual noise (e.g., Layton, 1975) mechanism may be contributing to the observed visual perception differences across age groups.

Summary

A limited sample of topics related to the initial registration and interpretation of visual stimuli was examined in this chapter. The topics ranged from absolute detection of light, to motion judgments, to jigsaw puzzle tasks of spatial integration. All are involved in some manner in the transformation of visual information into cognitive representations, and most of them have been found to decline somewhat with increased age. This clearly has important implications for the higher cognitive processes discussed in previous chapters since if the information is not adequately perceived it cannot be acquired, retained, comprehended, or utilized.

Physical changes in the optical characteristics of the visual system (e.g., decreased lens flexibility, reduced pupil size, increased opacity) can account for some of the basic sensory results, but there are not yet satisfactory explanations to account for the age differences observed in dynamic acuity, motion judgment, or any of the aspects of spatial perception. A slower rate of processing coupled with a prolonged persistence to previous stimulation may account for the age differences in critical fusion frequency and visual masking tasks.

9. Attentional Capacity and Processing Resources

Much of the early research that led to the development of contemporary cognitive psychology was concerned with investigating the limits of human abilities. These limits were clearly evident in tasks such as span of apprehension, absolute judgment, reaction time, and in a variety of dual-task situations where two activities had to be performed simultaneously. After the restrictions on maximal performance were well documented, theorists started speculating as to the type of mechanisms that might be responsible for such limitations. Judging from its longevity, one of the most popular of the mechanisms proposed was a limit on the human's attentional capacity or processing resources. There is considerable confusion about the exact nature of attentional capacity, but all theorists agree that whatever it is, less of it leads to poorer performance on a variety of tasks.

As an example of some of the controversy surrounding the current usage of the attentional capacity and processing resources terms, the following questions are among the issues still hotly debated by researchers in the field. (1) Are the limits observed in certain situations a true reflection of scarce attentional capacity, or can they be explained simply as an undeveloped skill? (2) Is there a single pool of capacity, or are there separate capacities for different types of processes? (3) Does the total amount of capacity remain fixed, or can it vary across tasks and situations? And, (4) when capacity is allocated to more than one task, is some reserved for executive monitoring operations or is it all distributed and made available for actual task performance?

The existence of such fundamental questions indicates that there is presently poor understanding, or at least poor consensus, about the nature of attentional capacity or processing resources. This state of uncertainty has important implications for research on individual and developmental differences since if there is little agreement as to what capacity is, there can be even less agreement as to how it can be measured. Moreover, without some means of measuring the amount of capacity or resources available, these concepts take on a rather metaphysical quality and are of limited usefulness for purposes of explanation. Nevertheless, phrases such as "reduced processing resources" or "diminished attentional capacity" are appearing with increasing frequency in discussions of aging phenomena, and it is therefore desirable to examine the history and limitations of these concepts before reviewing the aging literature considered relevant to these notions.

History of the Capacity Concept

The idea of a limit in capacity being responsible for one's maximum level of performance can be traced to communication theory and the development of abstract measures of information. Scientists working with physical communication devices proposed that biological organisms might also be considered information transmitting or processing systems, and hence should be found to be limited in the amount of information that could be transmitted in a manner analogous to the restrictions imposed by the physical dimensions of communication channels. The only hindrance to the application of this perspective seemed to be the lack of a general measure of what was transmitted in biological systems. However abstract measures of information soon became available in which information was defined in terms of reduction of uncertainty (i.e., one bit of information was equivalent to 50% reduction in uncertainty), and optimism grew about the potential for information-processing analyses of human performance.

One of the first psychological applications of concepts from information and communication theory involved determination of the human channel capacity for transmitting information. This was done by examining the functional relationships between the amount of input to the organism and the amount of output subsequently produced in a variety of simple tasks. For example, the individual might be instructed to assign specific responses to a series of unidimensional stimuli varying only in size, and then to provide the appropriate response upon presentation of a given stimulus. A typical finding in this type of absolute judgment task was that the number of items correctly identified mirrored the number of items presented up to some limit, after which performance was essentially the same regardless of the number of different stimuli that were presented. Figure 9.1 illustrates this prototypical result. The point at which the output of the system fails to keep pace with

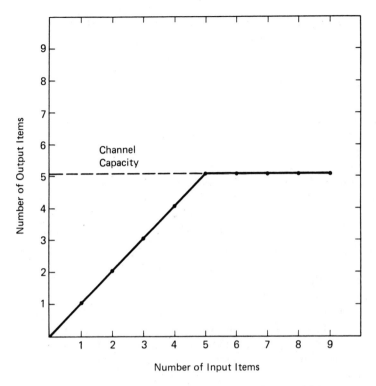

Figure 9.1. Determination of channel capacity as the point at which the number of correct output items fails to correspond to the number of input items.

increases in the input is considered to reflect the channel capacity of the system, in this case the human observer, for that type of information.

While there was considerable success in producing functions such as that portrayed in Figure 9.1 for tasks ranging from apprehension span to absolute judgment to immediate memory span, a number of problems soon became apparent. One of these was that the abstract information measure failed to account for the fact that many of the errors committed were only partially incorrect. That is, the information theory measure was restricted to absolute categories of correct or incorrect, and consequently it did not adequately reflect the partial information that was being transmitted when errors could be of differential severity. Some mistakes were very similar to the input message whereas others were completely dissimilar, and yet this distinction was ignored with the formal information measure.

A more important problem was evident in research on the span of immediate memory. Here it was discovered that it was not the formal information content of the material that was critical in determining the limits of memory, but rather the number of meaningful "chunks" into which the information could be organized. For example, words carry much more formal information than single letters, and yet we are generally able to remember as many unrelated words as unrelated letters. This type of result eventually led to the abandonment of the formal uncertainty-reduction concept of information, although the term information is still used to refer in a rather vague way to whatever it is that is processed by biological systems.

Despite these kinds of problems, the early application of information theory in psychology did lead to the development of a fairly specific conceptualization of capacity. According to this perspective, capacity was a structural limitation of the processing system essentially equivalent to the number of distinct mental states, or memory locations, that could be simultaneously activated when performing some task.

Somewhat later a dynamic measure of capacity was derived to measure throughput rate, or the amount of information transmitted per unit of time. A prototypical procedure for measuring information-processing rate involves presenting a number of stimuli that are below the capacity limit determined from static assessments, requiring that the responses be made as rapidly as possible, and then recording the interval elapsing between each stimulus and response. In this manner a graph could be constructed in which response time was plotted as a function of amount of input information (or actual information transmitted if there were errors in responding). The slope of the function represents time per unit of information, and consequently its reciprocal could be used as an estimate of dynamic capacity, or information processed per unit of time. As an example, consider two conditions involving two and four equally likely stimuli, respectively. Reaction time might average 300 msec in the condition with two stimuli, and 350 msec in the condition with four stimuli. Since the amount of information is 1 bit with two stimuli and 2 bits with four stimuli, the information transmission rate would be the reciprocal of the slope, i.e., $1/[(350-300)/(2-1)]$, or .02 bits/msec.

Unfortunately, this dynamic measure of capacity also was found to be inadequate as a number of experimental results appeared indicating that the slope of the information-time function was much reduced, sometimes even to a value of 0, by extensive practice or high degrees of stimulus-response compatibility. Since the reciprocal of the slope was assumed to be a reflection of capacity, these results led to the implication that capacity could be increased, perhaps to an infinite amount, by various experimental manipulations. This was obviously an unacceptable conclusion, and therefore the interpretation of capacity as amount of information transmitted per unit time has also been generally abandoned by recent researchers.

Although these early conceptualizations of capacity based on information theory measures are no longer accepted, they have resulted in a legacy of two general perspectives towards the concept of capacity; one structural and static, the other rate-related and dynamic. This structural-dynamic distinction is roughly analogous to the different ways one might speak of the capacity of a banquet hall as opposed to the capacity of a fast food restaurant. In the case of the banquet hall one is primarily interested in the total number of seats available in order to assess the maximum number of diners that can be accommodated at one time. However, with a fast food restaurant it is probably more meaningful to speak of capacity in terms of the number of that can be served in a given period of time. A similar distinction is often made when referring to the capacity of computers. On the one hand there is the memory or structural capacity consisting of the total amount of information accessible to the computer; on the other hand there is dynamic capacity in terms of the amount of information that can be handled in a limited period of time.

The structural-dynamic distinction is not without its problems, e.g., in some computers the memory states have to be continuously refreshed such that the dynamic capacity or processing rate can determine the number of active memory locations, but it seems useful as a general framework for categorizing research procedures and explanations concerned with attentional capacity or processing resources.

Usages of the Capacity Concept

Capacity and resource concepts have been increasingly employed as "explanations" for age differences observed in a variety of situations. For example, it is well known that memory performance can be improved by greater organization, mediation, and elaboration. It has also been discovered that older adults typically engage less often or less effectively in such beneficial processes compared to young adults. In order to explain why these processes decrease in effectiveness or frequency with increased age it is sometimes suggested that the resources necessary for carrying out those processes are diminished as one grows older in adulthood (e.g., see the discussion of effortful and automatic processing in Chapter 7).

This type of explanation, in which an age-related reduction in the amount of some unspecified capacity is assumed to be responsible for whatever cognitive differences are observed between young and old adults, is obviously not very meaningful without some independent means of assessing the total amount of capacity available to an individual. Primarily explanatory usages of capacity or resource concepts will therefore not be of concern here, and instead the focus will be on attempts either to document, or to measure the amount of, age-related reductions in capacity or resources.

Single-Task Procedures

The most direct means of determining an individual's capacity for processing simply involves the presentation of a task at several systematically manipulated levels of difficulty. The logic is similar to that illustrated in Figure 9.1, which is actually a special case of the more general procedure. An individual's capacity is inferred from the difficulty level (represented on the abscissa) at which performance decrements (portrayed on the ordinate) first become obvious. The units would be specific to the manner in which task difficulty was manipulated, but some generality might be obtained by carrying out similar procedures with a variety of different tasks.

It is rather surprising that very few studies have apparently utilized this procedure in comparisons of young and old adults. One of the reasons may have been a recognition that capacity and resource interpretations are not particularly useful in this context because of the absence of additional converging operations. Our understanding of the relevant mechanisms is not substantially improved by attributing the observed performance limitations to a restriction in amount of attentional capacity or processing resources since a number of other interpretations are just as plausible and often considerably more meaningful. For example, absolute-judgment and perceptual-span tasks may be limited by peripheral, sensory (structural) factors rather than amount of processing resources. Determination of the quantitative limits of perform-ance across ages in a variety of different tasks may therefore have little theoretical importance, but such data could be useful in human-factors applications and therefore it is unfortunate that more information of this type is not available.

Dual-Task Procedures

Probably the greatest application of capacity and resource concepts in contemporary cognitive psychology is in situations where two activities are performed simultaneously. A common finding is that performance on one or both tasks is degraded relative to the level of performance achieved when the tasks are performed separately. This dual-task or divided-attention decrement is often interpreted as indicating that the demands of the two concurrent tasks exceed the attentional capacity or processing resources available to the individual. Each task is assumed to require a finite amount of capacity or resources when performed alone, and together the sum of the requirements may be greater than the total amount available and therefore cause perform-ance to be impaired on one or both tasks. Although seldom explicitly stated, this type of reasoning seems to be based upon a static or structural concep-tualization of attentional capacity.

It is primarily on the basis of aging studies employing two concurrent tasks that led Burke and Light (1981) to make the following statement:

> A well-established finding in research on aging is that the elderly have diminished processing capacity in that they are less able than are the young to divide attention between two tasks to be performed simultaneously. (pp. 528–529)

However, we will soon see that this conclusion is based on an inadequate empirical foundation, and that all interpretations based on dual-task para-digms must be considered cautiously because of the number of questionable assumptions involved with this procedure.

At first impression it might appear that the dual-task procedure could easily be used to quantify an individual's capacity for attention, or resources for processing. All that seems necessary is to have two tasks with unambiguous performance measures, and to have the capability of systematically manipulating the difficulty (capacity requirements) of at least one of the tasks. The difficulty level at which performance decrements are evident on one or both tasks could serve as an estimate of attentional capacity.

Limitations of the Dual-Task Procedure. Unfortunately, while the preceding sequence of steps is plausible, no less than five distinct types of problems have been discovered that greatly complicate interpretations from the dual-task procedure. Many of these problems relate to the assumption that there is a single fixed pool of general capacity, and that the only cause of impaired performance is processing demands exceeding available capacity. For example, one objection to the dual-task logic is that interference with two concurrent tasks can arise from sources other than a limited processing capacity. Two tasks might compete for the same processing "structures," and therefore joint performance would be impaired because the relevant structures could only be used for one activity at a time. An extreme illustration might be the simultaneous performance of writing and typing with one's right hand. Because these two tasks require the same physical structure (i.e., the right hand) for their output, performance on one or both tasks will be degraded relative to the single-task situation even if the demands are considerably below the available capacity for attention. Only if this type of structural interference is ruled out, e.g., by demonstrating no performance impairment at low levels of task difficulty in the dual-task situation, can one make capacity interpretations of performance decrements with two simultaneous activities.

A second objection to the type of reasoning proposed above is that there is not yet convincing evidence that the amount of capacity remains constant in all situations, or that there is only one source of capacity rather than a number of structure-specific capacities. At least one theorist (Kahneman, 1973) has explicitly rejected a fixed limit on capacity and instead argued that the amount of capacity available depends upon situational and motivational factors. If it is true that the amount of attentional capacity allocated to tasks is variable, then it will obviously be difficult if not impossible to obtain a reasonable estimate of the total amount. There is also considerable debate as to whether capacity is unitary and relevant to all processes, or whether each process has its own source of capacity. Only in the former case will the interpretations of dual-task impairments as reflections of limitations on capacity be meaningful. One could still hope to assess the amount of capacity within each separate structural pool, but this is much more complicated as the requirements by various tasks on each pool of capacity are not known and overall task performance could be affected by demands exceeding any one of the several different capacities.

A third objection is that while the procedure for estimating total capacity may be reasonable if performance on one of the tasks remains the same in single- and dual-task situations, in practice it is often found that both tasks exhibit performance decrements in the dual-task situation. The difficulty in this case is that the two tasks might have quite different resource demands such that witholding the same amount of capacity leads to a performance reduction of, for example, two units in task A and only one unit in task B. This problem can be solved, but it requires the generation of complete performance operating characteristic functions (e.g., Norman & Bobrow, 1975; Sperling & Melchner, 1978) in which performance on task A is plotted against performance on task B across several conditions involving different relative emphases on the two tasks. Such a function provides a direct assessment of the value of units in one task in terms of units of the other task. Time-sharing decrements can then be determined by reference to the shape of the performance operating characteristic, or by an analysis of the area of the region bounded by the minimum and maximum performance levels on each task subsumed under the performance operating characteristic (Somberg & Salthouse, in press). Unless some procedure of this type is carried out it is impossible to make precise quantitative comparisons of the degree of impairment, or the amount of capacity expended, when performance is degraded on two dissimilar concurrent tasks.

Another problem with the reasoning from dual-task procedures is that it is not clear that all of the available capacity would be directly allocated to the tasks since it is conceivable that a sizable fraction might be held in reserve to handle the special requirements of two concurrent activities. Some theorists (e.g., Norman & Bobrow, 1975) assume that the available capacity is completely divided across two concurrent tasks, but others (e.g., Moray, 1967; Taylor, Lindsay, & Forbes, 1967) have argued that a portion of the capacity is needed for overhead, i.e., executive or control functions. At present there is little empirical evidence to distinguish between these alternatives, and thus it is quite possible that estimates of amount of capacity could be very misleading if the overhead requirements vary across tasks, situations, or individuals.

A fifth objection to using the dual-task procedure to make inferences about the amount of available capacity is that some tasks can apparently be performed without placing demands upon the hypothesized capacity. There may be a variety of reasons for this capacity independence, e.g., the task may be limited by the quality of the data rather than the amount of resources (Norman & Bobrow, 1975), the task might be automatic as a consequence of long practice (Shiffrin & Schneider, 1977), or the tasks might be grouped with one another such that no more total capacity is required to perform the tasks in combination than separately (Kantowitz, 1974). Regardless of the reason, if one or both tasks do not require capacity for their performance it is not appropriate to use dual-task procedures to assess available capacity.

A reasonable number of experimental studies have been reported in which dual-task procedures were administered to groups of young and old adults, but all studies suffered from one or more of the problems just described and therefore it is not yet possible to derive satisfactory measures of the amount of processing resources available to adults of different ages. The various studies differed in their respective limitations, however, and therefore it is instructive to examine why each is inadequate for making inferences about age differences in processing capacity.

Dichotic Listening. The most commonly employed dual-task procedure with adults of varying ages has been the dichotic-listening paradigm in which a series of items, typically digits, are simultaneously presented to each ear and the listener is instructed to recall as many items as possible from each ear in a designated sequence. Dichotic listening can be considered a dual-task situation if the input into each ear is assumed to represent a separate task. Inferences about processing capacity in the dichotic listening paradigm might be obtained by assuming that the two tasks (inputs to the two ears) are formally identical, and thus the sum of their performances can serve as an estimate of total capacity utilization in the dual-task (dichotic) situation. An estimate of the capacity required in the single-task situation can be derived by assuming that the traditional digit span, i.e., maximum recall of digits presented binaurally to both ears, reflects total capacity. Comparisons of these two estimates of processing capacity can therefore provide information about the relative amounts of capacity expended in single- and dual-task conditions, and the difference can be interpreted as an index of the cost of having to divide one's attention.

Data allowing an analysis of this type are available in reports by Inglis and Caird (1963) and Inglis and Ankus (1965). Both experiments included standard digit-span measures as well as dichotic presentations of from one to six digits in each ear. The data from the two extreme age groups in the Inglis and Caird (1963) experiment are plotted in Figure 9.2. (The Inglis and Ankus, 1965, data provide virtually identical results.) Three features of this figure are particularly interesting. First, note that the maximum level of summed performance in the dichotic situation (i.e., amount recalled from the right ear plus amount recalled from the left ear) is considerably less than the level of performance achieved in the standard digit span (which was the same for both young and old adults). This suggests either: (a) that some of the total capacity is required to monitor the special requirements of simultaneous presentation of material (e.g., rapid switching of an attentional "filter" from one ear to the other, or keeping track of which stimuli arrived in each ear); (b) that the amount of capacity allocated is variable, with apparently more distributed to the single digit-span task than to the dichotic task; or (c) that structural interference is responsible for the poorer performance with simultaneous presentations in the two ears.

It is also interesting that the difference between the capacity estimated from the digit span and the summed performance from the two dichotic tasks tends to increase with increases in the amount of input information. Consider only the group of young adults. The memory span was 6.3 digits, but the sum of

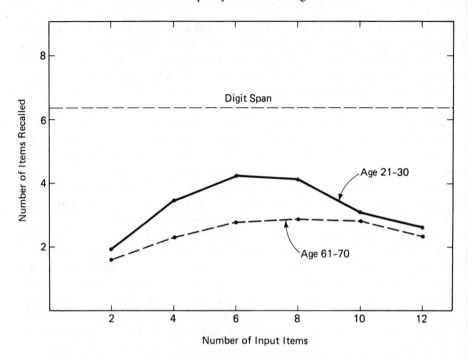

Figure 9.2. Single-task (digit span) and dual-task (dichotic listening) performance as a function of the number of input items. Both age groups had the same digit span but performed in the manner illustrated in the dichotic listening task. Data from Inglis and Caird (1963).

the items correct on the two ears was 4.23 for an input list of 6 (3 digits in each ear), 4.10 for an input list of 8, 3.08 for an input list of 10, and only 2.66 for an input list of 12. This complicates interpretations even further as it appears either that the amount of capacity allocated varies across different dual-task conditions as well as between single- and dual-task conditions, or that the amount of capacity required to handle the coordination of the two tasks increases with the difficulty of the component tasks. In any case, it seems clear that the dichotic-listening paradigm is not as simple as it initially appeared.

The third important feature of Figure 9.2 is that the older adults appear to exhibit the same general trends as the young adults, but are always at a lower level of performance. It is rather surprising that performance differences would be evident with only two and four input items (i.e., one or two digits per ear), as these should be well within everyone's capacity. Two possibilities to account for the age differences in the simplest conditions are that the older adults have some structural interference that the young adults do not, e.g., increased auditory impairment, or that more of the older adults' processing capacity is required for dual-task monitoring than that of younger adults.

These alternatives cannot be clearly distinguished at the present time, although the former alternative is supported by the Parkinson et al. (1980) finding that young and old adults screened for auditory sensitivity and matched on digit span do not differ in performance on dichotic-listening tasks.

To summarize, there are two important limitations of most of the research employing dichotic presentation. One is that the possibility of structural interference limiting performance in one or both age groups has not been ruled out, and therefore decrements in the dual-task situation cannot simply be attributed to limits on available capacity or resources. The second problem is that the data suggest that the amount of available capacity, or the proportion of capacity required for dual-task monitoring, may not be fixed across conditions and levels of task difficulty. As discussed earlier, it is impossible to determine the total amount of available capacity if that amount is not constant across various conditions. Therefore despite the numerous studies reporting age differences in dichotic listening situations (e.g., Craik, 1977, cited 10 separate studies), it must be concluded that this paradigm is not very useful for investigating possible age differences in the amount of available processing capacity.

Other Dual-Task Studies. Several other frequently cited dual-task studies are also inadequate for a variety of reasons. For example, an experiment by Kirchner (1958) required young (ages 18–24 years) and old (ages 60–84 years) adults to make keypress responses to stimulus lights under conditions in which the response was to the light physically present at that time, or to lights presented one, two, or three lights previously. The older adults were more affected than young adults by the requirement to respond to earlier presented stimuli, and many older participants were unable to even perform the task in the two- and three-back conditions. It is clear that the stimulus-response coding manipulation led to pronounced age differences, but without measures of single-task performance to provide a contrast for the dual-task performance it is impossible to quantify the amount of decrement in each age group.

A similar objection can be applied to an experiment by Broadbent and Heron (1962) in which young and old adults were compared in a digit-cancelling task and an auditory-monitoring task. There was no assessment of performance on the auditory-monitoring task when it was performed alone, and thus one cannot compare the magnitude of the time-sharing (i.e., dual-task vs. single-task) decrement across age groups. Older adults were slower and less accurate than the young adults in the dual-task condition but quantitative comparisons of amount of processing resources, or of the costs of divided attention, are simply not possible.

An experiment by Botwinick and Storandt (1974a) contrasted digit-span measures obtained under normal and "distracting" conditions, with the distraction consisting of repetitive finger tapping. Nearly the same estimates of digit-span were found in the two conditions for all age groups, thus suggesting that the tapping task was not sufficiently demanding of general capacity, or of the same type of specific capacity as that required for the digit-span task. With either alternative the negative results are not informative about the amount of capacity available to individuals in any age group.

Three studies have been reported in which performance was assessed in single- and dual-task situations for two tasks that both appeared to require capacity or resources. The first of these was an experiment by Talland (1962) in which young (early 20s) and older (ages 40–63 and 75–89 years) adults were required to perform two manual tasks separately and together. One of the tasks involved manipulating a counter, and the other consisted of using tweezers to pick up small colored beads. The older adults were poorer than the young adults on each task in both the single- and dual-task situations. This suggests that the older adults had greater difficulty in the time-sharing situation, but quantitative comparisons are impossible with such different tasks because performance operating characteristics were not derived. Also, because the two groups of adults differed in their performance in the single-task conditions, it could be argued that the dual-task condition merely added to the overall difficulty of each task and that older adults were more affected because they were already performing at a lower level in each component task.

A more recent experiment by Wright (1981) is subject to the same criticisms. Here the two tasks were a digit-span task and a verbal-reasoning task, and older adults were once again poorer in both tasks under single-task conditions. With six digits to be remembered the older adults (mean age of 68 years) recalled 88% correctly, while the young adults (mean age of 19 years) recalled 96%. The older adults in the corresponding condition of the reasoning task required about 5.97 sec to respond whereas the young adults responded in an average of 4.66 sec. (The experiment was actually quite complicated and a number of less demanding conditions were also employed but the important points can be illustrated in this single condition.)

Wright (1981) reported that older adults had greater performance decrements than the young adults with the added complexity of having to perform both tasks simultaneously. As with the Talland (1962) experiment, then, this result clearly indicates that the older adults experience greater problems with the more difficult dual-task situation. However, again it is impossible to quantify the amount of difficulty because the tasks were quite different and there was no performance operating characteristic generated to allow assessments of the "cost" of improved time or accuracy in one task by reduced performance in the other task.

The problem of separating general increases in task difficulty from unique requirements of the divided-attention situation was also considered by Wright (1981), and a second experiment demonstrated that similar increases in the performance differences between young and old adults could be obtained by simply manipulating the processing requirements in a single-task situation. Different manipulations were carried out in the two experiments and thus direct comparisons of dual-task and single-task increases in overall task complexity could not be conducted, but it is clear that the requirement to perform two simultaneous tasks is not the only manipulation that increases the magnitude of age differences in performance.

When two tasks, each having some nonzero level of difficulty, are performed concurrently, it is inevitable that the total difficulty or complexity of the joint task will be greater than either single task. It is therefore likely that the effects observed in many dual-task situations are no different than those that would be obtained when task difficulty or complexity is manipulated in a single task. This argument thus suggests that the requirement of performing two concurrent tasks is simply another means of increasing task complexity, and that there may not be a specific age deficit associated with divided attention, per se.

Two dual-task comparisons were examined in the context of a large project reported by Salthouse and Somberg (1982c), but mixed results were obtained and no definite conclusions are possible. One comparison involved a contrast between accuracy of detecting small targets in two visual arrays when they were presented successively, or simultaneously. Both young (mean age 23 years) and old (mean age 69 years) adults were less accurate with the simultaneous presentation, but the magnitude of the difference between successive and simultaneous conditions was the same across age groups and across 50 sessions of practice. This could be interpreted as indicating that the additional capacity required for the simultaneous (dual-task) condition was equally available to young and old adults, although it is possible that performance in the successive (single-task) condition was limited not by general capacity but by structural factors (i.e., the stimulus arrays were quite large and a sensory limitation of effective visual field may have been involved).

The second dual-task comparison available in the Salthouse and Somberg (1982c) report involved a vocal reaction time task performed either in isolation, or concurrently with a series of other perceptual-motor tasks. Performance on the other tasks was affected very little by the presence of the vocal reaction time task and thus the primary results are the reaction times in the single- and dual-task conditions. The older adults had a greater difference between the dual-task and single-task reaction time measures than did the young adults, and both groups tended to reduce these dual-task decrements with increased practice. Unfortunately the results are complicated by extremely large within-group variability, and the main effect of age on vocal reaction time was not statistically significant. It appears that the older adults had less reserve processing capacity than the young adults to devote to the vocal reaction time task, but the absence of expected age differences in the single-task reaction time measure indicates that other factors may also have been operating.

No definite conclusion about age differences in capacity can therefore be reached from the Talland (1962), Wright (1981), and Salthouse and Somberg (1982c) experiments. It seems that the age differences in performance increase when the difficulty of a task is increased by the requirement to perform another simultaneous activity, but in most cases the young adults were superior in the single-task condition and there was no provision for assessing the trade-offs in performance on the two concurrent tasks.

A recent experiment by Somberg and Salthouse (in press) was designed to determine whether age differences would be present in dual-task situations when the performance of young and old adults was equated in the single-task situation. This experiment was apparently also the only one to have compared complete performance operating characteristics in young and old adults. The two tasks both involved visual discrimination in order to minimize the possibility that different structural resource pools were involved in the performance of each task. These tasks also allowed initial performance to be equated by adjusting the duration of the visual displays in order that each research participant achieved between 80% and 90% accuracy when concentrating entirely on one task. In different conditions individuals were induced to vary the relative emphasis on each task, and thus complete performance operating characteristics could be constructed for each individual.

The principal finding in the Somberg and Salthouse experiment was that young (mean age 20 years) and old (mean age 65 years) adults had virtually identical performance operating characteristics. That is, once the two groups of individuals were equated for their initial level of performance, ability to divide attention across two different tasks was the same for young and old adults. Both age groups exhibited the same quantitative performance decrements, relative to their performance when concentrating entirely on a single task, when attempting to divide their attention between two tasks.

A second experiment in the same report (Somberg & Salthouse, in press) extended this finding with two manual tasks, one involving repetitive keying in a fixed sequence and the other auditory reaction time. Performance could not be directly equated across the two age groups in these tasks, but comparisons of dual-task performance relative to performance in the single-task conditions indicated that the young (mean age 19 years) and old (mean age 69 years) adults exhibited the same quantitative amount of decrement when performing two concurrent tasks. Griew (1958) had earlier reported a similar experiment, with a tracking rather than a keying task, and also found nearly identical time-sharing performance in two age groups. He used adults who did not differ very much in age (i.e., 24–31 years vs. 42–50 years) and consequently their performance levels were equivalent in the single-task conditions. More recently, Parkinson et al. (1980) reported that the age difference in dichotic-listening performance was eliminated by screening for auditory sensitivity and matching individuals of different ages on standard digit span.

Taken together, these experiments, particularly those of Somberg and Salthouse (in press), suggest that there is little age difference in divided attention per se, because adults of varying ages appear to perform identically when their initial level of performance is similar either because of duration adjustment, because of restricted age ranges, or because of matching of individuals. This conclusion conflicts with frequently repeated claims that divided-attention situations present particular problems for older adults (e.g., Burke & Light, 1981; Craik, 1977; Wright, 1981), but as discussed above, most of the evidence considered to support that position is far from definitive. It does seem reasonable to conclude that older adults are generally poorer than young adults at a variety of activities, and that increasing the difficulty of the activity will tend to affect the performance of older adults more than young adults. However, such a conclusion is not unique to the divided-attention situation, and direct attempts to investigate age differences in ability to allocate or divide one's attention have not revealed striking differences beyond what can be accounted for by base task differences.

None of the studies described in this section have been able to provide quantitative assessments of the amount of processing capacity available to an individual and therefore the major issue of whether there are age differences in amount of processing capacity has not been satisfactorily resolved with experiments using dual-task procedures.

Dynamic Measures of Capacity

The classical measure of information-processing rate in which the reciprocal of the slope of the function relating reaction time to stimulus information is interpreted as an estimate of dynamic processing capacity has been employed in a number of different studies with older adults. However, in addition to the problems with this measure discussed earlier (e.g., its dependency on state of practice and degree of stimulus-response compatibility), there has been an inconsistent pattern of results in the studies comparing information-transmission rate in adults of differing ages. Some experiments appear to indicate equivalent slopes for young and old adults (e.g., Crossman & Szafran, 1956; Goldfarb, 1941; Szafran, 1966, 1968), while others have revealed larger slope parameters for older adults (e.g., Griew, 1959b; 1964; Suci, Davidoff, & Surwillo, 1960).

One factor that may be contributing to this inconsistency is the grossness of the required response. The three studies reporting larger slopes in older adults involved simple (i.e., stylus release or vocal) responses, while Crossman and Szafran (1957) employed a card-sorting task and Goldfarb (1941) included both reaction and movement time in his measurements. Age differences in the slope parameter may not have been apparent with the more complicated responses because the greater time and variability may have hidden the small but systematic age effects. This explanation is not completely satisfactory as Szafran (1966, 1968) used relatively simple key-press responses, and an alternative post hoc interpretation to account for the discrepancies among these studies has been proposed by Welford (1977). However, in light of the interpretation problems, and the inconsistent results presently available, studies employing classical information theory procedures cannot be considered very useful with respect to the issue of possible age differences in processing capacity.

A procedure similar to that employed for measurement of information-transmission rate is Sternberg's (1969) memory-scanning paradigm in which reaction time to a probe stimulus is examined as a function of the number of items in the previously presented memory set. It was reported in Chapter 6 that older adults have steeper memory-scanning slopes (i.e., greater increases in reaction time with each additonal memory set item) than young adults (see Figure 6.2). The relationship between attentional capacity and the slope parameter in this paradigm is based on the finding that the slope reduces to a value approximating zero with moderate levels of practice on the task. This led to the interpretation (e.g., Shiffrin & Schneider, 1977) that the slope is a reflection of the amount of demands upon a fixed amount of processing capacity. With a moderate degree of experience the memory-scanning task presumably becomes automatic and requires less processing capacity, thereby accounting for the shallower slope after practice.

A functionally equivalent interpretation to account for individual differences in the slope parameter might postulate that the memory-scanning task at a given level of practice places the same absolute demands upon varying amounts of capacity, such that the slope can serve as an approximate index of the proportion of total capacity required by the task. With this perspective, therefore, the steeper slopes of older adults could be interpreted as indicating that there is a smaller amount of processing capacity available with increased age.

One problem with this capacity interpretation is that two recent studies have demonstrated that the age differences in the memory scanning slope parameter are much reduced or even eliminated with extensive practice (e.g., Plude & Hoyer, 1981; Salthouse & Somberg, 1982c). Both groups of researchers assumed that with practice the scanning task may have become automatic, and independent of capacity. However, if a factor such as experience can lead to capacity independence, one might question whether the individual differences evident at early stages of practice might also be attributable to various degrees of capacity independence. In other words, memory-scanning slope differences might reflect alternative degrees of reliance on the same fixed amount of capacity, rather than a fixed proportion of differing total amounts of capacity. At the present time these two alternatives do not appear to be empirically distinguishable.

Moreover, while the resource interpretation of the memory-scanning slope parameter is currently popular, it should also be noted that other interpretations are conceivable. For instance, two alternatives discussed by Salthouse and Somberg (1982c) were that shallower slopes could be a consequence of a different mode of processing (e.g., parallel rather than serial comparison), or a different organization of the stimulus items (e.g., separate memory set items could be coded or grouped into the same functional category). If either of these interpretations is eventually supported the speculations about capacity differences based on the larger slopes of older adults would obviously have to be rejected.

There is at least one additional technique that has been proposed to assess dynamic processing capacity based on reaction time measurements. This is the speed-accuracy tradeoff procedure in which instructions or payoffs are employed to encourage an individual to produce a range of reaction times at varying levels of accuracy. Since the slope of the function relating accuracy to reaction time represents the increase in accuracy (or stimulus information) achieved per unit of time, it has been interpreted (e.g., Swensson, 1972; Thomas, 1974) as a relatively pure measure of dynamic information-processing capacity.

Only two studies have reported direct age comparisons of the speed-accuracy slope parameter, and unfortunately the results were not very consistent. In the first study (Salthouse, 1979), different speed and accuracy values were obtained in separate blocks of trials, and a rather coarse procedure was used to derive slope estimates. In the later study (Salthouse & Somberg, 1982b) a complete range of speed-accuracy values was derived within a single trial block, and a more precise method of computing the slope was used in which values at chance and perfect levels of accuracy were eliminated for each individual prior to computing the regression parameters relating reaction time and accuracy.

Because the second study used more exact procedures and included larger sample sizes, its results are probably more meaningful. These were that young (mean age of 19 years) and old (mean age of 69 years) adults had virtually identical slopes, and only differed in the intercept parameter reflecting the reaction time at which accuracy began to improve above the chance level. This finding could be interpreted as indicating that there is no age difference in processing capacity defined as the amount of increase in information per unit of time. Such a conclusion must be very tentative at the present time, however, since the earlier study did find shallower slopes in some samples of older adults, and there is not yet any independent evidence that the slope of the speed-accuracy function is truly a valid reflection of processing capacity.

Conclusions about Age Differences in Capacity

The discussion of the preceding two sections indicates that there is presently little concrete evidence concerning adult age differences in attentional capacity or processing resources. A number of problems serve to complicate interpretations from experiments employing the dual-task technique, and it has been difficult to separate the unique requirements of division of attention from the increased difficulty associated with having to perform two activities rather than just one. Dynamic measures of capacity have also not fared well as the various procedures each have problems, and none have yielded unequivocal results.

Despite the frequency with which the resource and capacity terms have been used in the contemporary literature, it appears that very little can be definitely stated about these concepts. We are not yet able to measure this mystical entity, and therefore assertions about varying amounts or demands upon it are mere conjecture at the present time. Moreover, there have been very few attempts to relate the capacity and resource constructs to conceptually similar processes that have already been identified and investigated. For example, capacity from the structural perspective appears to be functionally equivalent to the span of immediate memory or to the size of primary or working memory. In this particular case the connection to an established concept may not prove very beneficial as there is still considerable confusion about the effects of increased age on primary memory capacity (see Chapter 7). Generally, however, there is a need to develop explicit ties to other theoretical and empirical phenomena, and to provide operational definitions of capacity and resources that allow one to estimate the amount available to a given individual in a specific task. The following section attempts to perform these functions with a dynamic conceptualization of capacity.

Processing Rate As an Alternative to Capacity

Although notions of capacity or resources are currently very popular in cognitive psychology theories, a mechanism that might prove more useful in characterizing individual differences, particularly those associated with adult age, is the rate of processing information. A slowing of most behavioral activities with increased age has been extremely well-documented (e.g., Salthouse, in press), and among the explanations proposed to account for this phenomenon is a slower speed of nearly all elementary operations within the nervous system. This class of explanation is not yet well accepted, although a recent review (Salthouse, in press) concluded that there is at least as much evidence for this position as any alternative interpretation that has been proposed to account for the slowing-with-age phenomenon.

The implications of the hypothesis that nearly every neural event takes somewhat longer in the older nervous system are widespread and dramatic (cf. Salthouse, 1980; Salthouse & Kail, in press). For example, consider two computers with different minimum cycle times. The slower computer will not only execute all programming operations at a slower rate, but if the external environment is changing or the internal memories are decaying, there will also be a greater probability of error in the slower system. A fundamental difference at such a basic level in the processing system would also lead to the expectation of a variety of procedural or strategic differences at higher levels of operation in order to compensate for the slower operation speed. (Indeed, given the unequivocal evidence that there are substantial age differences in the rate of processing information, the burden would seem to be on theorists proposing more complicated interpretations to demonstrate that age differences in internal processing rate could not be responsible for the effects that are observed.)

Figure 9.3 illustrates in a very gross fashion how variations in processing rate might lead to such higher-level differences. Input from the environment are designated as stimulus events because the individual typically has limited control over their sequence and duration. The processing operations are unlabeled in order to allow generality across a variety of different types of tasks. For example, in problem-solving situations the operations might correspond to: A—understanding the problem statement; B—focusing on relevant details; C—considering alternative conceptualizations; and D—formulating tentative solutions. In memory tasks the operations might reflect: A—stimulus registration; B—superficial encoding; C—rehearsal; and D—elaboration and association with previous information. Spatial integration tasks in perception might involve the operations of: A—perception of one

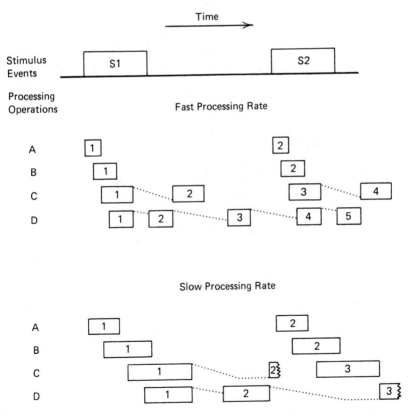

Figure 9.3. Illustration of how a difference in rate of processing internal information could lead to both quantitative and qualitative changes in performance. See text for details.

segment; B—perception of a second segment; C—examination of the relation-ship between segments; and D—formation of a tentative hypothesis about the whole figure.

No claim is made that these tasks are necessarily performed in exactly the manner illustrated. In fact, the particular operations involved and the sequence in which they are carried out is actually irrelevant for the present argument. All that is necessary is that various activities involve processing operations which each require time, and that by a mechanism such as decay or interference the products of at least some of those operations decrease in availability over a period of time (represented by the dotted lines below certain operations).

Several consequences of a slower processing rate are evident in Figure 9.3. First, notice that because of the longer time for each operation, performance with a slow processing rate will be more dependent upon the pacing of external events than with a fast rate of processing. Some operations (e.g., C2) may not be completed at even relatively slow presentation rates, and many more operations would suffer at faster stimulus paces. Also observe that what may be the most important operations will tend to suffer the most with a slower processing rate because they are dependent upon the products of earlier operations. The key to successful task performance may be repetitive appli-cation of an operation (e.g., D) that is dependent upon the successful completion of earlier operations (e.g., B and C). If the rate of performing the primitive operations is slower there will be fewer opportunities for the critical operation to be performed. In behavioral terms these aspects may be mani-fested in the absolute magnitude of age differences increasing directly with the number or complexity of the operations involved in the task, i.e., an interaction between age and task complexity.

It is also apparent in Figure 9.3 that variations in processing rate might have important consequences even when there is no external control on the time of stimulus or response. Products of earlier operations (e.g., the dotted lines originating from C1 and D2) might be needed for later operations (e.g., C2, D3), but if the time intervening between these operations is too great the necessary information may no longer be available. This will be manifested as a reduction in performance accuracy or quality even though the primary cause was actually a slower rate of processing. Indeed with complex processes the operation of the processing rate mechanism may not be recognizable because the primary changes it produces have led to the development of secondary effects such as the utilization of different modes of operation or the employ-ment of alternative task strategies.

The preceding discussion has been fairly abstract because there is not yet much agreement as to what specific operations are involved in various cognitive tasks. Nonetheless, it should be clear that whatever the nature of these operations, the rate at which they are completed will likely have important consequences at many levels of processing.

Similar speculations about the potential importance of age differences in the speed of elementary operations have been offered for many years, as evidenced by the following quote from Jones (1956):

> ... in any mental task which requires relative judgments about external events while they are still in progress it is necessary to integrate data which are received at rates which may not be within the subject's control. As observation slows down, failure begins to occur at difficulty levels which were formerly met successfully. A similar principle may apply in any thought process in which the subject must make successive comparisons and reach judgments based on ongoing series of mental events. When the results of these comparisons emerge too slowly, the level of effective problem-solving declines, primarily because the earlier steps in the series are lost before the new integrations are achieved. (p. 138)

Birren (e.g., 1956, 1965, 1974) has also been a long and strong advocate of the importance of speed in age differences in behavior, but the processing-rate perspective has still not received serious consideration in theoretical interpretations of aging phenomena. Despite its long-standing neglect, the processing-rate hypothesis has the advantage of providing a single mechanism to account for an extremely diverse set of results, and unlike the capacity concept, processing rate might be operationally defined with fairly simple tasks such as choice reaction time or time to escape visual backward masking. Considerable work remains to be done to determine how various measures of processing rate interrelate with one another, and how rate of processing affects various cognitive operations. However, the very solid empirical foundation for the hypothesis that speed of processing becomes slower with increased age, coupled with the realization that a difference at such an elementary level would have profound consequences at many higher levels of activity, indicates that this perspective warrants detailed investigation.

Theoretical Evaluation

There is virtually no empirical evidence in the literature on age differences in attentional capacity or processing resources that is directly relevant to the theoretical dimensions of maturation versus environment, performance versus competence, and general versus specific. Most researchers working in this area probably assume that maturational factors are responsible for any capacity differences that might be postulated, but in the absence of relevant data environmental determinants cannot be ruled out. There is currently much controversy in the mainstream research on attention about whether there are situational or individual differences in the efficiency of allocating one's capacity (i.e., whether allocation reflects performance or competence), and whether there is a single general capacity or multiple specific capacities, and thus there is clearly no conclusion possible with respect to how these factors are affected by aging.

The processing-rate interpretation of age differences in cognitive perform-ance is closely related to the neural noise theory discussed in Chapter 3 and thus it would be classified as maturational, competence-based, and general in application.

Summary

One of the most pervasive "explanations" of age differences in cognitive performance, perhaps second only to "cohort effects," is that there is an age-related reduction in the capacity or resources available for carrying out cognitive activities. The idea of capacity limitations in human performance has had a brief but active history in experimental psychology and it is not surprising that this concept would be incorporated into interpretations of adult age differences. Unfortunately, there is presently little agreement as to what capacity is, and no satisfactory method for measuring its amount or quantity.

Dual-task procedures are faced with a number of interpretation problems, and the available evidence suggests that increased overall difficulty or com-plexity rather than the requirement of having to share one's attention among several simultaneous activities is responsible for most of the age differences in divided-attention situations. Alternative attempts at defining capacity have also not been markedly successful, and for none is there any validity information indicating that capacity or resources are truly being measured.

One of the more promising of the attempts to find a unitary explanation for a variety of observed age differences substitutes processing rate for capacity or resources. This conceptualization has the advantage of an already estab-lished empirical data base, and an operational definition of the basic concept, i.e., processing rate might be measured with tasks such as choice reaction time. It is probably unrealistic to expect that an explanation based on a single mechanism will be found to be applicable in many different contexts, but the processing-rate interpretation appears to have remarkable generality at the present time.

10. Speculations and Implications

This final chapter contains no new discussions of research findings, but instead presents speculations about the practical and theoretical implications of the research reviewed in previous chapters. There are four main sections, with the first consisting of a summary of the best-documented age trends reported in earlier chapters. The second section contains a discussion of the practical significance of these laboratory results, and the third an examination of issues confronting the development of a satisfactory functional age assessment device. The fourth section concludes with an evaluation of the current state of theoretical development in cognitive aging.

Five Major Age Trends

A very extensive body of literature concerned with age differences in cognitive processes has been reviewed in the preceding chapters, and in order to provide a brief overview it is desirable to abstract out a limited number of processes for which there is unequivocal evidence of age differences. The following list represents such a capsule summary, although it must be recognized that any grouping of this type is necessarily arbitrary as less, more, or different, categories could easily be justified.

It should also be pointed out that while there can be little doubt about the age-related decline in the abilities listed, no firm statements can be made about the relative rates of decline. The available data are generally inadequate to quantify the magnitude of the age trend because of small samples or too few age groups, and because the available dependent variables provide an ability index at only a single level of difficulty.

Reasoning and Decision Making

On the basis of the psychometric tests of reasoning reviewed in Chapter 4 (i.e., the series-completion and Raven's Progressive Matrices tests), and the variety of decision-making aspects examined in Chapter 5 (e.g., creativity, flexibility, etc.), it can be concluded that increased age is often associated with a decline in the efficiency, and perhaps the effectiveness, of reasoning and decision-making processes.

Memory

A great variety of memory tasks reviewed in Chapter 7 indicate that older adults are less proficient than young adults at remembering many types of information. It also appears that the age differences are especially pronounced when the to-be-remembered material can be organized or elaborated to facilitate integration with existing knowledge.

Spatial Abilities

An age-related decline in spatial abilities was first noted in the psychometric tests reviewed in Chapter 4, and elaborated in the examination of analysis, integration, and manipulation skills in Chapter 8.

Perceptual-Motor and Cognitive Speed

The dramatic age trends in the WAIS Digit Symbol Substitution Test reported in Chapter 4 indicate that speeded processes are impaired with increased age, and the results from temporal perception tasks reviewed in Chapter 8 further confirm this conclusion. It is also likely that internal cognitive processes are affected by the slowing and not just input (perceptual) and output (motor) processes, as both the rate of memorial activation and rehearsal have been found to be slower with increased age.

Sensory Factors

Although there has been little explicit discussion of sensory processes in the present monograph, the brief mention of this topic in Chapter 8 indicates that there are substantial age differences in sensory processes concerned with the detection and discrimination of environmental information.

In addition to these five specific categories of age differences, there also appears to be a fairly consistent trend for the absolute magnitude of the performance differences between age groups to increase directly with task complexity (see pages 142 and 189). This phenomenon is extremely important since the extent to which any specific process appears to be age-sensitive may be determined by the difficulty (processing requirements) of a task, almost regardless of the nature of the activity.

Taken together, the five categories of specific processes and the general tendency of age differences to be proportional to overall task complexity present an imposing, and rather depressing, picture of the cognitive effects of aging. Increased age in adulthood seems to be a disadvantage in most laboratory tests of cognitive processes. In fact, an argument could be made that the observed age differences are even more remarkable when considered in the context of the widely varying experiences people have during adulthood. Life experiences are fairly uniform in the childhood years due to the dependency upon adults and nearly universal school attendance, but as adults there is great diversity in occupation, leisure activity, and residential style. Discovering systematic effects of age in the midst of such experiential variability clearly attests to the potency of age-related factors.

Some observers have become quite alarmed at the pessimistic image of older adults suggested by these types of results and have almost apologetically sought more optimistic interpretations. For example, despite an absence of compelling evidence, there is an amazing amount of enthusiasm for suggestions that the reported age differences are simply due to motivational factors, to sensory or muscular weaknesses, or to unspecified "cohort" effects. While it is unlikely that such simplistic interpretations will find broad support, it is probably true that the existing research literature does not present a completely accurate picture of the true capabilities of older adults. Cognitive processes in which there is not an age decrement, or possibly even an age increment, are not well represented in the research literature and consequently cannot be summarized here.

At least two factors contribute to the absence of more encouraging results about cognitive aging in the scientific literature. One factor is what has been termed "prejudice against the null hypothesis," or the reluctance to consider as meaningful a finding of no differences between groups or conditions. In other words, a finding of differences between age groups has been considered inherently more interesting than a finding of no differences, and consequently results indicating a decline in an ability have been more likely to appear in the published literature than results suggesting age stability. This type of bias may be disappearing with an increase in sophistication about statistical power since it is now possible for investigators to demonstrate that their procedures (i.e., sample sizes and observed variability) had a reasonable probability of detecting a difference of a given magnitude had it really existed.

A second factor contributing to the underrepresentation of age-stable or age-increment functions in the research literature is that many of the processes that improve with experience, and hence with age in most cases, have been difficult to study in the laboratory. Wisdom, sagacity, and judgment are

202 10. Speculations and Implications

examples of abilities often assumed to improve with age or experience, but which have thus far proven difficult or impossible to examine in a rigorous, scientific fashion. These abilities are extremely complex, and it may be many years before even a primitive understanding of them is available. Until that time, however, it must be realized that the existing research may not be providing a completely accurate perspective of the capabilities of older adults.

Practical Significance

A hope was expressed in Chapter 1 that an examination of the cognitive effects of aging might help identify the impact upon society of a progressively older population. The discovery that age has adverse effects on a number of cognitive processes such as those summarized in the preceding section clearly provides an initial step in the direction of determining the consequences of aging on an individual's functioning in society. In light of the results described in previous chapters, the age trends reported in Chapter 1 concerning professional achievement, industrial performance, and automobile driving seem quite reasonable. Indeed, if the laboratory findings are considered valid, one is struck by the remarkable *absence* of age effects in most normal activities. People over the age of 50 or 60 are not noticeably deficient in their daily activities at home or on the job, and older adults are generally quite competent at self-care, arranging transportation, coping with changing regulations and environmental conditions, etc. To some extent, therefore, it becomes necessary to explain why the age effects that are so dramatic in laboratory measures are not also evident in the behaviors of everyday life. Four likely explanations are discussed below.

Probably one of the major reasons why the performance of daily activities is not noticeably affected by increased age is that the variations across individuals of the same age level are typically so enormous that even fairly large age differences may be overlooked. For example, very few of the age functions illustrated in the previous chapters have revealed age differences as large as 50%, but it is not uncommon to find differences of this magnitude among individuals from the same age range. Age differences might therefore be present in daily activities but are simply difficult to detect without systematically controlled observations.

A second possibility is that the laboratory tasks may actually be irrelevant to the skills of daily living, and that they are merely measuring trivial aspects of behavior that are not important in normal functioning. This is a difficult objection to deal with because it may always be possible to think of a specific individual who appears not to use a particular type of ability, and thus there may be an element of truth to this assertion. For the most part, however, this objection can be dismissed because an explicit goal of much of cognitive psychology has been to investigate processes relevant to daily life, and there is presently no evidence that the processes isolated in laboratory investigations are not those involved in extralaboratory activities. It is probably the case that there are still other processes relevant to daily activities that have not yet been investigated by cognitive psychologists (cf. Neisser, 1976), but without further information it is unreasonable to claim that those that have been examined are completely irrelevant to "real-world" functioning. The linkage from laboratory to real life is by no means firmly established, but the hypothesis that laboratory tasks bear no relationship to normal activities is presently without empirical foundation.

A third possibility to account for the absence of dramatic age differences in normal tasks is that most of the activities of daily living are only minimally demanding, such that they can be performed by even the least competent individuals. Therefore even if there is a decline with age in some of the components of those abilities, it is still likely that most people will have enough in reserve to handle nearly all normal situations. An implication of this view is that while age differences might not be evident in typical activities, they may become apparent if some type of unusual stress or complication is present as is often the case in laboratory tasks. As an example, the physiological functioning of older adults may be superficially indistinguishable from that of young adults in moderate climates, but the older adults are more likely to exhibit dramatic reactions to extreme hot or cold temperatures because they are physiologically less efficient at internal temperature regulation. An analogous situation may exist in the cognitive domain as age differences may not be evident under normal, undemanding circumstances, but may become much more obvious when the task or environment becomes more complex and stressful.

The fourth possibility that might explain why more dramatic age differences have not been noted in the performance of the activities in one's home and place of employment is that these tasks have been highly practiced for literally thousands of hours. Very little is presently known about how experience changes the nature of a skill, but it is obvious that regardless of the specific mechanisms eventually discovered experience leads to dramatic improvements in the efficiency and effectiveness of performance. Since increased age in adulthood is generally positively correlated with experience, many highly practiced activities may be maintained at a constant level despite age-related declines in component ability because of the compensating effects of greater experience. Indeed the important question for many activities may be the age at which the increase in experience fails to exceed, or keep pace with, the decline in the component processes.

It should be clear that there is not yet a good understanding of the practical significance of the age differences that have been observed in cognitive functioning. The four factors discussed above undoubtedly contribute to this situation, but probably the greatest hindrance to knowledge about the relationships between laboratory performance and extralaboratory competence is simply lack of detailed information about the nature of real-world activities (cf. Fozard & Popkin, 1978; Hartley, Harker, & Walsh, 1980). Cognitive psychologists have made reasonable progress in identifying a limited number of basic processes or operations thought to be responsible for the performance of different laboratory tasks, although there is admittedly little evidence documenting that the same processes are involved in what appear to be related tasks. What is markedly deficient, however, is adequate knowledge about the specific processes involved in various real-world activities. Until detailed job analyses are conducted one must be content to rely on speculation and intuition in attempting to relate laboratory findings to extralaboratory situations. According to this reasoning, then, the failure to predict the practical implications of the observed age differences is not attributable to problems inherent in adult cognitive psychology, but rather to inadequate understanding of the specific requirements of actual jobs—the normal province of industrial psychology. Of course switching the locus of responsibility from one subdiscipline to another does not resolve the issues, but it does suggest that a redistribution of research resources might prove profitable for assessing the practical implications of many research findings.

Prospects for Functional Age Measurement

The preceding discussion concerning the possibility of experience partially or completely compensating for age-related ability declines implies that abstract functional age measures will probably not be suitable for determining an individual's competency in a professional or industrial situation. Because the individual will likely have developed task-specific skills and strategies while working on the job, the results from a set of rather abstract tasks cannot be a substitute for direct assessments of actual work proficiency. Heron and Chown (1967) reached a similar conclusion in summarizing the findings of their study of functional age: "The functions which are of interest in a particular situation should be tested in their own right and performance assessed on these" (p. 137). Although functional age measures will probably not solve the problems concerned with determining an individual's overall competency, they can still be very useful for a variety of other applications (e.g., vocational selection, health assessment, stress evaluation). It is therefore desirable to examine some of the issues that should be considered when attempting to construct a viable functional age battery.

At least three fundamental questions must be resolved before one can attempt to construct a reasonable assessment device to measure functional age. One basic question concerns the type of tests to be employed—either existing psychometric tests that are already standardized and of known reliability, or specially devised tests modified from laboratory cognitive tasks.

The disadvantage of the former is that the measures obtained from most existing psychometric tests are not theoretically meaningful (i.e., easily interpretable) from the perspective of contemporary cognitive psychology in that they involve uncertain mixtures of a number of different cognitive processes. As noted above, there are not yet direct ties between cognitive laboratory tasks and real-life activities. However, when such relationships are established it is likely that they will be strongest when examined at the level of elementary cognitive processes such as those isolated in cognitive laboratory tasks rather than the complicated combinations of processes found in psychometric tests. The disadvantage of the use of specially constructed tests is that the procedures will have to be standardized for easy administration, and large-scale studies will have to be conducted to ensure that the measures are of adequate reliability.

A second basic question concerns the selection of the ability dimensions to be assessed—the ability categories or factors can be determined by an intuitively based organizational scheme, or by a large-scale factor analysis. It is naturally much easier to categorize according to abilities which seem to be involved in the various tests, but one's intuitions may be quite wrong such that tests grouped within the same ability category are actually independent or that tests placed in different categories are closely related. The much more complicated factor analysis technique, although requiring substantial data and statistical analysis, minimizes the likelihood of these types of errors. This technique involves administering a large number of candidate tests from several different ability domains to very large samples of adults, and then examining the pattern of correlations from the matrix of individuals and tests to determine the degree of relationship between, and within, ability groupings.

A third issue to be considered when selecting tests for the functional age battery is whether the primary criterion is age sensitivity or behavioral representativeness. If the former criterion is emphasized only tests known to exhibit substantial age effects would be included, and although the battery might be very accurate in predicting an individual's relative position on the derived age function, it may be completely useless for predicting performance on any nonlaboratory activity. The latter criterion would obviously reverse these weightings, with improved real-life predictability but at the cost of reduced accuracy of "pure-age" localization.

The present discussion of functional age measurement is primarily intended to provide some cautions concerning the premature development and application of a functional age battery. It is almost certainly possible to select a set of sensory and cognitive tasks that would allow fairly accurate prediction of an individual's chronological age, but the validity of such tasks would remain questionable without better understanding of the activities performed by that individual. The development of a truly useful functional age battery must therefore await better specification of the nature of the cognitive processes involved in real-world activities, and further development of job analyses from a cognitive perspective.

Theoretical Assessment

While the preceding sections have indicated that there is considerable knowledge about the types of cognitive differences that exist between young and old adults, and that there is beginning to be an awareness of the practical implications of these differences, it must be concluded that there is very little basis for optimism concerning the current level of theoretical understanding of adult age differences in cognition. Three extremely broad dimensions for theory classification and two illustrative theories representing polar extremes along each dimension were introduced in Chapter 3, and at the end of all subsequent chapters results relevant to each dimension were considered and the theoretical positions evaluated. Almost without exception these theoretical evaluations revealed that the absence of relevant data made definite conclusions impossible at the present time. This is truly a discouraging reflection on the existing state of research because the theoretical dimensions were explicitly selected to represent major and fundamental, rather than subtle and trivial, issues. Nevertheless, there is still very little convincing evidence that allows definitive localization along any of the dimensions, and neither the disuse nor the neural noise type of theory can yet be unequivocally rejected.

Some of the lack of progress in theoretical understanding may be attributable to a tendency among most cognitive researchers in aging to focus on small-scale, limited-scope interpretations of specific phenomena while ignoring the sizable age differences reported in other related areas. It is probably unrealistic to expect all age differences to be subsumed within a single theoretical perspective, but it is also true that the number of explanations need not equal the number of aging phenomena that have been discovered. Many cognitive processes may be determined by the same fundamental age-related mechanisms, and lack of awareness of the nature of age differences in other related processes may unnecessarily restrict the generality and usefulness of theoretical interpretations.

As an example, hypotheses in memory and aging have been largely derived from theoretical perspectives developed in research on young adults, and consequently much of the research has focused on investigating age effects in theoretical processes such as interference, organization, retrieval, etc. While these efforts have provided many useful facts, it is important not to forget that the ultimate goal is to develop an explanation of age differences in all cognitive processes and not just one specific aspect of memory. Greater overall progress might therefore be achieved by considering age differences in, for example, creativity and flexibility of problem solving, in the analysis, integration, and manipulation of spatial information, and in the speed of registration, comprehension, and integration of information, when proposing interpretations of age-related phenomena in any given topic area.

In an earlier paper (Salthouse, 1980) it was argued that most contemporary researchers working in adult cognition have relied exclusively on the strategy of generating hypotheses from theories developed in the mainstream of psychology. Alternative strategies for selecting hypotheses are to derive them from theories in the field of aging, or from the established empirical phenomena dealing with aging. Either of these latter strategies would likely lead to better integration of theoretical interpretations across various subareas in adult cognition.

Recognizing that aging likely produces a variety of related cognitive changes and that research hypotheses can derive from sources other than mainstream psychology may also shift the focus from description (*which* processes are age sensitive?) to explanation (*why* are these processes affected by age?). It was mentioned in Chapter 3 that a disadvantage of the "borrowing from the mainstream" strategy is that no mechanism is typically available to explain why the relevant process is different with increased age. Awareness of the age trends evident in related processes may lead to the identification of a primary age mechanism that is responsible for a variety of cognitive effects.

The preceding comments should not be interpreted to mean that unitary or monolithic mechanisms must be incorporated into all theoretical explanations, but merely that theorists working in this area might profit from an awareness of the broader context in which one's own results must be placed. However, the temptation is too great not to mention one final time that the processing-rate interpretation is not subject to the criticisms raised above in that it appears to provide a single mechanism with sufficient generality to account for a great variety of age-related cognitive differences.

Summary

The present summary will be quite brief because the chapter itself can be considered a summary of the preceding chapters. These chapters have clearly revealed that there are a number of cognitive processes in which substantial age-related declines exist. The relationships of these laboratory findings to natural activities is still tenuous, largely because of an inadequate understanding of the component processes involved in real-world endeavors. It was argued that the development of a functional age assessment battery is probably premature at this time, although a number of issues that must be considered in the eventual development of such a battery were discussed. The lack of substantial theoretical progress was deplored, and a proposal offered for remedying this situation.

References

Abrahams, J.P., Hoyer, W.J., Elias, M.F., & Bradigan, B. Gerontological research in psychology published in The Journal of Gerontology 1963–1974: Perspectives and progress. *Journal of Gerontology,* 1975, *30,* 668–673.

Adam, J. Statistical bias in cross-sequential studies of aging. *Experimental Aging Research,* 1977, *3,* 325–333.

Adam, J. Sequential strategies and the separation of age, cohort, and time-of-measurement contributions to developmental data. *Psychological Bulletin,* 1978, *85,* 1309–1316.

Adamowicz, J.K. Visual short-term memory and aging. *Journal of Gerontology,* 1976, *31,* 39–46.

Adamowicz, J.K. Visual short-term memory, age, and imaging ability. *Perceptual and Motor Skills,* 1978, *46,* 571–576.

Adamowicz, J.K., & Hudson, B.R. Visual short-term memory, response delay, and age. *Perceptual and Motor Skills,* 1978, *46,* 267–270.

Alpaugh, P.K., & Birren, J.E. Variables affecting creative contributions across the adult life span. *Human Development,* 1977, *20,* 240–248.

Amberson, J.L., Atkeson, B.M., Pollack, R.H., & Malatesta, V.J. Age differences in dark-interval threshold across the life span. *Experimental Aging Research,* 1979, *5,* 423–433.

Anastasi, A. *Differential Psychology.* New York: MacMillan, 1958.

Anders, T.R., & Fozard, J.L. Effects of age upon retrieval from primary and secondary memory. *Developmental Psychology,* 1973, *9,* 411–415.

Anders, T.R., Fozard, J.L., & Lillyquist, T.D. Effects of age upon retrieval from short-term memory. *Developmental Psychology,* 1972, *6,* 214–217.

Annett, M. The classification of instances of four common class concepts by children and adults. *British Journal of Educational Psychology,* 1959, *29,* 223–236.

Arenberg, D. Anticipation interval and age differences in verbal learning. *Journal of Abnormal Psychology*, 1965, *70*, 419–425.

Arenberg, D. Age differences in retroaction. *Journal of Gerontology*, 1967, *22*, 88–91. (a)

Arenberg, D. Regression analyses of verbal learning on adult age at two anticipation intervals. *Journal of Gerontology*, 1967, *22*, 411–414. (b)

Arenberg, D. Concept problem solving in young and old adults. *Journal of Gerontology*, 1968, *23*, 279–282. (a)

Arenberg, D. Input modality in short-term retention of old and young adults. *Journal of Gerontology*, 1968, *23*, 462–465. (b)

Arenberg, D. A longitudinal study of problem solving in adults. *Journal of Gerontology*, 1974, *29*, 650–658.

Arenberg, D. The effects of input condition on free recall in young and old adults. *Journal of Gerontology*, 1976, *31*, 551–555.

Arenberg, D. The effects of auditory augmentation on visual retention for young and old adults. *Journal of Gerontology*, 1977, *32*, 192–195.

Arenberg, D. Differences and changes with age in the Benton Visual Retention Test. *Journal of Gerontology*, 1978, *33*, 534–540.

Arenberg, D. Estimates of age changes on the Benton Visual Retention Test. *Journal of Gerontology*, 1982, *37*, 87–90.

Arvey, R.D., & Mussio, S.J. Test discrimination, job performance, and age. *Industrial Gerontology*, 1973 (Winter), 22–29.

Atkeson, B.M. Differences in magnitude of simultaneous and successive Mueller-Lyer illusions from age twenty to seventy-nine years. *Experimental Aging Research*, 1978, *4*, 55–66.

Attig, M., & Hasher, L. The processing of frequency of occurrence information by adults. *Journal of Gerontology*, 1980, *35*, 66–69.

Axelrod, S., & Cohen, L.D. Senescence and embedded figure performance in vision and touch. *Perceptual and Motor Skills*, 1961, *12*, 283–288.

Bacon, F. *The Essays or Counsels, Civil and Moral.* New York: Odyssey Press, 1937. (Originally published in 1620).

Bahrick, H.P. Maintenance of knowledge: Questions about memory we forgot to ask. *Journal of Experimental Psychology: General*, 1979, *108*, 296–308.

Bahrick, H.P., Bahrick, P.O., & Wittlinger, R.P. Fifty years of memory for names and faces: A cross-sectional approach. *Journal of Experimental Psychology: General*, 1975, *104*, 54–75.

Balinsky, B. An analysis of mental factors of various age groups from nine to sixty. *Genetic Psychology Monographs*, 1941, *23*, 192–234.

Baltes, P.B. Longitudinal and cross-sectional sequences in the study of age and generation effects. *Human Development*, 1968, *11*, 145–171.

Baltes, P.B., Cornelius, S.W., Spiro, A., Nesselroade, J.R., & Willis, S.L. Integration versus differentiation of fluid/crystallized intelligence in old age. *Developmental Psychology*, 1980, *16*, 625–635.

Baltes, P.B., & Goulet, L.R. Exploration of developmental variables by manipulation and simulation of age differences in behavior. *Human Development*, 1971, *14*, 149–170.

Baltes, P.B., & Labouvie, G.V. Adult development of intellectual performance: Description, explanation, and modification. In C. Eisdorfer & M.P. Lawton (Eds.),

The Psychology of Adult Development and Aging. Washington, D.C.: American Psychological Association, 1973.

Baltes, P.B., Nesselroade, J.R., Schaie, K.W., & Labouvie, E.W. On the dilemma of regression effects in examining ability-level-related differentials in ontogenetic patterns of intelligence. *Developmental Psychology,* 1972, *6,* 78–84.

Baltes, P.B., Reese, H.W., & Nesselroade, J.R. *Life-span Developmental Psychology: Introduction to Research Methods.* Monterey, Calif.: Brooks/Cole, 1978.

Baltes, P.B., & Schaie, K.W. The myth of the twilight years. *Psychology Today,* 1974, *8,* 35–40.

Baltes, P.B., & Schaie, K.W. On the plasticity of intelligence in adulthood and old age: Where Horn and Donaldson fail. *American Psychologist,* 1976, *31,* 720–725.

Baltes, P.B., & Willis, S.L. Toward psychological theories of aging and development. In J.E. Birren & K.W. Schaie (Eds.), *Handbook of the Psychology of Aging.* New York: Van Nostrand Reinhold, 1977.

Barclay, R., & Comalli, P.E. Age differences in perceptual learning on the Mueller-Lyer Illusion. *Psychonomic Society,* 1970, *19,* 323–325.

Barrett, T.R., & Wright, M. Age-related facilitation in recall following semantic processing. *Journal of Gerontology,* 1981, *36,* 194–199.

Bartlett, J.C., & Snelus, P. Life-span memory for popular songs. *American Journal of Psychology,* 1980, *93,* 551–560.

Basowitz, H., & Korchin, S.J. Age differences in the perception of closure. *Journal of Abnormal and Social Psychology,* 1957, *54,* 93–97.

Bayley, N., & Owen, M.H. The maintenance of intellectual ability in gifted adults. *Journal of Gerontology,* 1955, *10,* 91–107.

Bearison, D. The construct of regression: A Piagetian approach. *Merrill-Palmer Quarterly,* 1974, *20,* 21–30.

Beeson, M.F. Intelligence at senescence. *Journal of Applied Psychology,* 1920, *4,* 219–234.

Belbin, E., & Downs, S. Activity learning and the older worker. *Ergonomics,* 1964, *7,* 429–438.

Belbin, E., & Downs, S. Interference effects from new learning: Their relevance to the design of adult training programs. *Journal of Gerontology,* 1965, *20,* 154–159.

Bell, B. Retinal field shrinkage, age, pulmonary function, and biochemistry. *Aging and Human Development,* 1972, *3,* 103–109.

Bell, B., Wolf, E., & Berholz, C.D. Depth perception as a function of age. *Aging and Human Development,* 1972, *3,* 77–81.

Belmore, S.M. Age-related changes in processing explicit and implicit language. *Journal of Gerontology,* 1981, *36,* 316–322.

Berg, C., Hertzog, C.K., & Hunt, E. Age differences in the speed of mental rotation. *Developmental Psychology,* 1982, *18,* 95–107.

Berger, L., Bernstein, A., Klein, E., Cohen, J., & Lucas, G. Effects of aging and pathology on the factorial structure of intelligence. *Journal of Consulting Psychology,* 1964, *28,* 199–207.

Berkowitz, B. The Wechsler-Bellevue performance of white males past age 50. *Journal of Gerontology,* 1953, *8,* 76–80.

Bilash, I., & Zubek, J.P. The effects of age on factorially "pure" mental abilities. *Journal of Gerontology,* 1960, *15,* 175–182.

Binet, A., & Henri, V. La psychologie individuelle. *L'Annee Psychologique,* 1895, *2,* 411–465.

Binet, A., & Simon, T. Methodes nouvelles pour le diagnostic due niveau intellectual des anormaux. *L'Annee Psychologique,* 1905, *11,* 191–244.

Birkhill, W.R., & Schaie, K.W. The effect of differential reinforcement of cautiousness in intellectual performance among the elderly. *Journal of Gerontology,* 1975, *30,* 578–583.

Birren, J.E. Age changes in speed of responses and perception and their significance for complex behavior. In *Old Age in the Modern World.* Edinburgh: Livingstone, 1955.

Birren, J.E. The significance of age changes in speed of perception and psychomotor skills. In J.E. Anderson (Ed.), *Psychological Aspects of Aging.* Washington, D.C.: American Psychological Association, 1956.

Birren, J.E. Principles of research on aging. In J.E. Birren (Ed.), *Handbook of Aging and the Individual.* Chicago: University of Chicago Press, 1959.

Birren, J.E. Age changes in speed of behavior: Its central nature and physiological correlates. In A.T. Welford & J.E. Birren (Eds.), *Behavior, Aging and the Nervous System.* Springfield, Ill.: Charles C Thomas, 1965.

Birren, J.E. Translations in Gerontology—From Lab to Life: Psychophysiology and speed of response. *American Psychologist,* 1974, *29,* 808–815.

Birren, J.E., Bick, M.W., & Fox, C. Age changes in the light threshold of the dark-adapted eye. *Journal of Gerontology,* 1948, *3,* 267–271.

Birren, J.E., & Botwinick, J. Rate of addition as a function of difficulty and age. *Psychometrika,* 1951, *16,* 219–232.

Birren, J.E., & Morrison, D.F. Analysis of the WAIS subtests in relation to age and education. *Journal of Gerontology,* 1961, *16,* 363–369.

Birren, J.E., & Renner, V.J. Research on the psychology of aging: Principles and experimentation. In J.E. Birren & K.W. Schaie (Eds.), *Handbook of the Psychology of Aging.* New York: Van Nostrand Reinhold, 1977.

Birren, J.E., Riegel, K.F., & Morrison, D.F. Age differences in response speed as a function of controlled variations of stimulus conditions: Evidence of a general speed factor. *Gerontologia,* 1962, *6,* 1–18.

Birren, J.E., Woods, A.M., & Williams, M.V. Behavioral slowing with age: Causes, organization, and consequences. In L.W. Poon (Ed.), *Aging in the 1980's.* Washington, D.C.: American Psychological Association, 1980.

Blackwell, O.M., & Blackwell, H.R. Visual performance data of 156 normal observers of various ages. *Journal of the Illuminating Engineering Society,* 1971, *1,* 3–13.

Blum, J.E. & Jarvik, L.F. Intellectual performance of octogenarians as a function of education and initial ability. *Human Ability,* 1974, *17,* 364–375.

Bogard, D.A. Visual perception of static and dynamic two-dimensional objects. *Perceptual and Motor Skills,* 1974, *38,* 395–398.

Botwinick, J. Perceptual organization in relation to age and sex. *Journal of Gerontology,* 1965, *20,* 224–227.

Botwinick, J. Disinclination to venture response versus cautiousness in responding: Age differences. *Journal of Genetic Psychology,* 1969, *115,* 55–62.

Botwinick, J. Behavioral processes. In S. Gershon & A. Raskin (Eds.), *Aging* (Volume 2). New York: Raven Press, 1975.

Botwinick, J. Intellectual abilities. In J.E. Birren & K.W. Schaie (Eds.), *Handbook of the Psychology of Aging.* New York: Van Nostrand Reinhold, 1977.

Botwinick, J. *Aging and Behavior.* New York: Springer, 1978.

Botwinick, J., & Arenberg, D. Disparate time spans in sequential studies of aging. *Experimental Aging Research*, 1976, *2*, 55–61.

Botwinick, J., & Brinley, J.F. Age differences in relations between CFF and apparent motion. *Journal of Genetic Psychology*, 1963, *102*, 189–194.

Botwinick, J., Brinley, J.F., & Robbin, J.S. Task alternation time in relation to problem difficulty and age. *Journal of Gerontology*, 1958, *13*, 414–417.

Botwinick, J., Robbin, J.S., & Brinley, J.F. Reorganization of perceptions with age. *Journal of Gerontology*, 1959, *14*, 85–88.

Botwinick, J., & Storandt, M. *Memory, Related Functions and Age*. Springfield, Ill.: Charles C Thomas, 1974. (a)

Botwinick, J., & Storandt, M. Vocabulary ability in later life. *Journal of Genetic Psychology*, 1974, *125*, 303–308. (b)

Botwinick, J., & Storandt, M. Recall and recognition of old information in relation to age and sex. *Journal of Gerontology*, 1980, *35*, 70–76.

Botwinick, J., West, R., & Storandt, M. Qualitative vocabulary test responses and age. *Journal of Gerontology*, 1975, *30*, 574–577.

Bowles, N.L., & Poon, L.W. The effect of age on speed of lexical access. *Experimental Aging Research*, 1981, *7*, 417–425.

Bransford, J.D., & Franks, J.J. The abstraction of linguistic ideas. *Cognitive Psychology*, 1971, *2*, 331–350.

Brebner, J. The effect of age on judgments of length. *Journal of Gerontology*, 1962, *17*, 91–94.

Breen, L.Z., & Spaeth, J.L. Age and productivity among workers in four Chicago companies. *Journal of Gerontology*, 1960, *15*, 68–70.

Brinley, J.F. Cognitive sets, speed, and accuracy of performance in the elderly. In A.T. Welford & J.E. Birren (Eds.), *Behavior, Aging and the Nervous System*. Springfield, Ill.: Charles C Thomas, 1965.

Brinley, J.F., & Fichter, J. Performance deficits in the elderly in relation to memory load and set. *Journal of Gerontology*, 1970, *25*, 30–35.

Brinley, J.F., Jovick, T.J., & McLaughlin, L.M. Age, reasoning and memory in adults. *Journal of Gerontology*, 1974, *29*, 182–189.

Broadbent, D.E. *Decision and Stress*. New York: Academic Press, 1971.

Broadbent, D.E., & Gregory, M. Some confirmatory results on age differences in memory for simultaneous stimulation. *British Journal of Psychology*, 1965, *56*, 77–80.

Broadbent, D.E., & Heron, A. Effects of a subsidiary task upon performance involving immediate memory by younger and older subjects. *British Journal of Psychology*, 1962, *53*, 189–198.

Bromley, D.B. Some experimental tests of the effects of age on creative intellectual output. *Journal of Gerontology*, 1956, *11*, 74–82.

Bromley, D.B. Some effects of age on short-term learning and remembering. *Journal of Gerontology*, 1958, *13*, 398–406.

Bromley, D.B. Age differences in the Porteus Maze Test. *Proceedings of the Seventh International Congress of Gerontology*, 1966, 225–228.

Bromley, D.B. Age and sex differences in the serial production of creative conceptual responses. *Journal of Gerontology*, 1967, *22*, 32–42.

Bromley, D.B. *The Psychology of Human Ageing*. Middlesex, England: Penguin, 1974.

Brown, C.W., & Ghiselli, E.E. Age of semiskilled workers in relation to abilities and interests. *Personnel Psychology*, 1949, *2*, 497–511.

Brozek, J., & Keys, A. Changes in flicker-fusion frequency with age. *Journal of Consulting Psychology*, 1945, *9*, 87–90.

Bruce, P.R., Coyne, A.C., & Botwinick, J. Adult age differences in metamemory. *Journal of Gerontology*, 1982, *37*, 354–357.

Bruning, R.H., Holzbauer, I., & Kimberlin, C. Age, word imagery, and delay interval: Effects on short-term and long-term retention. *Journal of Gerontology*, 1975, *30*, 312–318.

Burg, A. Visual acuity as measured by dynamic and static tests. *Journal of Applied Psychology*, 1966, *50*, 460–466.

Burg, A. Light sensitivity as related to age and sex. *Perceptual and Motor Skills*, 1967, *24*, 1279–1288.

Burg, A. Lateral visual field as related to age and sex. *Journal of Applied Psychology*, 1968, *52*, 10–15.

Burke, D.M., & Light, L.L. Memory and aging: The role of retrieval processes. *Psychological Bulletin*, 1981, *90*, 513–546.

Burton, A., & Joel, W. Adult norms for the Watson-Glaser Tests of Critical Thinking. *Journal of Psychology*, 1945, *19*, 43–48.

Buschke, H. Two stages of learning by children and adults. *Bulletin of the Psychonomic Society*, 1974, *2*, 392–394.

Buss, A.R. An extension of developmental models that separate ontogenetic changes and cohort differences. *Psychological Bulletin*, 1973, *80*, 466–479.

Buss, A.R. Methodological issues in life-span developmental psychology from a dialectical perspective. *International Journal of Aging and Human Development*, 1979, *10*, 121–164.

Caird, W.K. Aging and short-term memory. *Journal of Gerontology*, 1966, *21*, 295–299.

Campbell, D.P. A cross-sectional and longitudinal study of scholastic abilities over twenty-five years. *Journal of Counseling Psychology*, 1965, *12*, 55–61.

Canestrari, R.E. Paced and self-paced learning in young and elderly adults. *Journal of Gerontology*, 1963, *18*, 165–168.

Canestrari, R.E. The effects of commonality on paired associate learning in two age groups. *Journal of Genetic Psychology*, 1966, *108*, 3–7.

Canestrari, R.E. Age changes in acquisition. In G.A. Talland (Ed.), *Human Aging and Behavior*. New York: Academic Press, 1968.

Cattell, J. McK. Mental tests and measurements. *Mind*, 1890, *15*, 373–380.

Ceci, S.J., & Tabor, L. Flexibility and memory: Are the elderly really less flexible? *Experimental Aging Research*, 1981, *7*, 147–158.

Cerella, J., Paulshock, D., & Poon, L.W. The effects of semantic processing on memory of subjects differing in age. *Educational Gerontology*, 1982, *8*, 1–7.

Cerella, J., Poon, L.W., & Fozard, J.L. Mental rotation and age reconsidered. *Journal of Gerontology*, 1981, *36*, 620–624.

Cerella, J., Poon, L.W., & Fozard, J.L. Age and iconic read-out. *Journal of Gerontology*, 1982, *37*, 197–202.

Chance, J., Overcast, T., & Dollinger, S.J. Aging and cognitive regression: Contrary findings. *Journal of Psychology*, 1978, *98*, 177–183.

Chapanis, A. Relationships between age, visual acuity, and color vision. *Human Biology*, 1950, *22*, 1–31.

Charles, D.C. Comments on papers of Labouvie, Hoyer, and Gottesman. *Gerontologist*, 1973, *13*, 36–38.

Charman, D.K. The ageing of iconic memory and attention. *British Journal of Social and Clinical Psychology*, 1979, *18*, 257–258.

Charness, N. Components of skill in bridge. *Canadian Journal of Psychology*, 1979, *33*, 1–16.

Charness, N. Aging and skilled problem solving. *Journal of Experimental Psychology: General*, 1981, *110*, 21–38. (a)

Charness, N. Search in Chess: Age and skill differences. *Journal of Experimental Psychology: Human Perception and Performance*, 1981, *7*, 467–476. (b)

Charness, N. Visual short-term memory and aging in chess players. *Journal of Gerontology*, 1981, *36*, 615–619. (c)

Chown, S.M. Age and the rigidities. *Journal of Gerontology*, 1961, *16*, 353–362.

Christian, A.M., & Paterson, D.G. Growth of vocabulary in later maturity. *Journal of Psychology*, 1936, *1*, 167–169.

Cicirelli, V.G. Categorization behavior in aging subjects. *Journal of Gerontology*, 1976, *36*, 676–680.

Clark, L.E., & Knowles, J.B. Age differences in dichotic listening performance. *Journal of Gerontology*, 1973, *28*, 173–178.

Clay, H.M. A study of performance in relation to age at two printing works. *Journal of Gerontology*, 1956, *11*, 417–424. (a)

Clay, H.M. An age difficulty in separating spatially contiguous data. *Journal of Gerontology*, 1956, *11*, 318–322. (b)

Cohen, G. *The Psychology of Cognition.* New York: Academic Press, 1977.

Cohen, G. Language comprehension in old age. *Cognitive Psychology*, 1979, *11*, 412–429.

Cohen, G. Inferential reasoning in old age. *Cognition*, 1981, *9*, 59–72.

Cohen, J. The factorial structure of the WAIS between early adulthood and old age. *Journal of Gerontology*, 1957, *21*, 283–290.

Colavita, F.B. *Sensory Changes in the Elderly.* Springfield, Ill.: Charles C Thomas, 1978.

Cole, S. Age and scientific performance. *American Journal of Sociology*, 1979, *84*, 958–977.

Comalli, P.E., Wapner, S., & Werner, H. Perception of verticality in middle and old age. *Journal of Psychology*, 1959, *47*, 259–266.

Comfort, A. Test battery to measure ageing rate in man. *Lancet*, 1969 (Dec. 27), 1411–1415.

Conrad, H.S. General information, intelligence, and the decline of intelligence. *Journal of Applied Psychology*, 1930, *14*, 592–599.

Coppinger, N.W. The relationship between critical flicker frequency and chronological age for varying levels of stimulus brightness. *Journal of Gerontology*, 1955, *10*, 48–52.

Coren, S., & Porac, C. A new analysis of life-span age trends in visual illusion. *Developmental Psychology*, 1978, *14*, 193–194.

Corsini, R.J., & Fasset, K.K. Intelligence and aging. *Journal of Genetic Psychology*, 1953, *83*, 249–264.

Corso, J.F. *Aging Sensory Systems and Perception.* New York: Praeger, 1981.

Coyne, A.C. Age differences and practice in forward visual masking. *Journal of Gerontology*, 1981, *36*, 730–732.

Coyne, A.C., Eiler, J.M., Vanderplas, J.M., & Botwinick, J. Stimulus persistence and age. *Experimental Aging Research*, 1979, *5*, 263–270.

Coyne, A.C., Herman, J.F., & Botwinick, J. Age differences in acoustic and semantic recognition memory. *Perceptual and Motor Skills*, 1980, *51*, 439–445.

Craik, F.I.M. The nature of the age decrement in performance on dichotic listening tasks. *Quarterly Journal of Experimental Psychology*, 1965, *17*, 227–240.

Craik, F.I.M. Short-term memory and the aging process. In G.A. Talland (Ed.), *Human Aging and Behavior*. New York: Academic Press, 1968.

Craik, F.I.M. Applications of signal detection theory to studies of ageing. *Interdisciplinary Topics in Gerontology*, 1969, *4*, 147–157.

Craik, F.I.M. Age differences in recognition memory. *Quarterly Journal of Experimental Psychology*, 1971, *23*, 316–323.

Craik, F.I.M. Age differences in human memory. In J.E. Birren & K.W. Schaie (Eds.), *Handbook of the Psychology of Aging*. New York: Van Nostrand Reinhold, 1977.

Craik, F.I.M., & Masani, P.A. Age differences in the temporal integration of language. *British Journal of Psychology*, 1967, *58*, 291–299.

Craik, F.I.M., & Masani, P.A. Age and intelligence differences in coding and retrieval of word lists. *British Journal of Psychology*, 1969, *60*, 315–319.

Craik, F.I.M., & Simon, E. Age differences in memory: The roles of attention and depth of processing. In L.W. Poon, J.L. Fozard, L.S. Cermak, D. Arenberg & L.W. Thompson (Eds.), *New Directions in Memory and Aging*. Hillsdale, N.J.: Lawrence Erlbaum Associates, 1980.

Crook, M.N., Alexander, E.A., Anderson, E.M.S., Coules, J., Hanson, J.A., & Jeffries, N.T. *Age and Form Perception*. Randolph A.F.B., Texas: USAF School of Aviation Medicine, 1958.

Crook, M.N., Devoe, D.B., Hageman, K.C., Hanson, J.A., Krulee, G.K., & Ronco, P.G. *Age and the Judgment of Collison Courses*. Randolph A.F.B., Texas: USAF School of Aviation Medicine, 1957.

Crossman, E.R.F.W., & Szafran, J. Changes with age in the speed of information-intake and discrimination. *Experientia Supplementum IV: Symposium on Experimental Gerontology*. Basel: Birkhauser, 1956.

Cunningham, W.R., & Birren, J.E. Age changes in human abilities: A 28-year longitudinal study. *Developmental Psychology*, 1976, *12*, 81–82.

Cunningham, W.R., & Birren, J.E. Age changes in the factor structure of intellectual abilities in adulthood and old age. *Educational and Psychological Measurement*, 1980, *40*, 271–290.

Cunningham, W.R., Clayton, V., & Overton, W. Fluid and crystallized intelligence in young adulthood and old age. *Journal of Gerontology*, 1975, *30*, 53–55.

Cunningham, W.R., Sepkoski, C.M., & Opel, M.R. Fatigue effects on intelligence test performance in the elderly. *Journal of Gerontology*, 1978, *33*, 541–545.

Danziger, W.L. & Salthouse, T.A. Age and the perception of incomplete figures. *Experimental Aging Research*, 1978, *4*, 67–80.

Davies, A.D.M. Age and Memory For Designs Test. *British Journal of Social and Clinical Psychology*, 1967, *6*, 228–233.

Davies, A.D.M. Measures of mental deterioration in aging and brain damage. In S.M. Chown & K.F. Riegel (Eds.), *Psychological Functioning in the Normal Aging and Senile Aged*. Basel: Karger, 1968.

Davies, A.D.M., & Laytham, G.W.H. Perception of verticality in adult life. *British Journal of Psychology*, 1964, *55*, 315–320.

Davies, A.D.M., Spelman, M.S., & Davies, M.G. Combining psychometric data on brain damage and the influence of aging. *Perceptual and Motor Skills*, 1981, *52*, 583–592.

De La Marre, G., & Shepard, R.D. Ageing: Changes in speed and quality of work among leather cutters. *Occupational Psychology*, 1958, *32*, 204–209.

Demming, J.A., & Pressey, S.L. Tests indigenous to the adult and older years. *Journal of Consulting Psychology*, 1957, *4*, 144–148.

Denney, D.R., & Denney, N.W. The use of classification for problem solving; a comparison of middle and old age. *Developmental Psychology*, 1973, *9*, 275–278.

Denney, N.W. Clustering in middle and old age. *Developmental Psychology*, 1974, *10*, 471–475.

Denney, N.W. Task demands and problem solving strategies in middle-aged and older adults. *Journal of Gerontology*, 1980, *35*, 559–564.

Denney, N.W., & Denney, D.R. The relationship between classification and questioning strategies among adults. *Journal of Gerontology*, 1982, *37*, 190–196.

Denney, N.W., & Lennon, M.L. Classification: A comparison of middle and old age. *Developmental Psychology*, 1972, *7*, 210–213.

Denney, N.W., & Palmer, A.M. Adult age differences on traditional and practical problem-solving measures. *Journal of Gerontology*, 1981, *36*, 323–328.

Dennis, W. Age and achievement: A critique. *Journal of Gerontology*, 1956, *11*, 331–333.

Dennis, W. The age decrement in outstanding scientific contributions: fact or artifact? *American Psychologist*, 1958, *13*, 457–460.

Dennis, W. The long-term constancy of behavior: sentence length. *Journal of Gerontology*, 1960, *15*, 195–196.

Dennis, W. Creative productivity between the ages of 20 and 80 years. *Journal of Gerontology*, 1966, *21*, 1–8.

DeSilva, H.R. Age and highway accidents. *Scientific Monthly*, 1938, *47*, 536–545.

Desroches, H.F., Kaiman, B.D., & Ballard, H.T. Relationships between age and recall of meaningful material. *Psychological Reports*, 1966, *18*, 920–922.

Dewey, J. Introduction. In E.V. Cowdry (Ed.), *Problems of Ageing*. Baltimore: The Williams & Wilkins Co., 1939.

DiLollo, V. Temporal integration in visual memory. *Journal of Experimental Psychology: General*, 1980, *109*, 75–97.

DiLollo, V., Arnett, J.L., & Kruk, R.V. Age-related changes in rate of visual information processing. *Journal of Experimental Psychology: Human Perception and Performance*, 1982, *8*, 225–237.

Dirken, J.M. *Functional Age of Industrial Workers*. Groningen: Wolters-Noordhoff, 1972.

Dixon, R.A., Simon, E.W., Nowak, C.A., & Hultsch, D.F. Text recall in adulthood as a function of level of information, input modality, and delay interval. *Journal of Gerontology*, 1982, *37*, 358–364.

Doppelt, J.E., & Wallace, W.L. The performance of older people on the Wechsler Adult Intelligence Scale. *American Psychologist*, 1955, *10*, 338–339.

Drachman, D.A., & Leavitt, J. Memory impairment in the aged: Storage vs. retrieval. *Journal of Experimental Psychology*, 1972, *93*, 302–308.

Edwards, A.E., & Wine, D.B. Personality changes with age; their dependency on concomitant intellectual decline. *Journal of Gerontology*, 1963, *18*, 182–184.

Eisdorfer, C., Axelrod, S., & Wilkie, F.L. Stimulus exposure time as a factor in serial learning in an aged sample. *Journal of Abnormal and Social Psychology*, 1963, *67*, 594–600.

Eisner, D.A. Life-span age differences in visual perception. *Perceptual and Motor Skills*, 1972, *34*, 857–858.

Elias, C.S., & Hirasuna, N. Age and semantic and phonological encoding. *Developmental Psychology*, 1976, *12*, 497–503.

Elo, A.E. Age changes in master chess performance. *Journal of Gerontology*, 1965, *20*, 289–299.

Erber, J.T. Age differences in recognition memory. *Journal of Gerontology*, 1974, *29*, 177–181.

Erber, J.T. Age differences in learning and memory on a digit-symbol substitution task. *Experimental Aging Research*, 1976, *2*, 45–53.

Erber, J.T. Age differences in a controlled-lag recognition memory task. *Experimental Aging Research*, 1978, *4*, 195–205.

Erber, J.T., Herman, T.G., & Botwinick, J. Age differences in memory as a function of depth of processing. *Experimental Aging Research*, 1980, *6*, 341–348.

Eriksen, C.W., Hamlin, R.M., & Breitmeyer, R.G. Temporal factors in visual perception as related to aging. *Perception and Psychophysics*, 1970, *7*, 354–356.

Eriksen, C.W., Hamlin, R.M., & Daye, C. Aging adults and rate of memory scan. *Bulletin of the Psychonomic Society*, 1973, *1*, 259–260.

Eriksen, C.W., & Steffy, R.A. Short-term memory and retroactive interference in visual perception. *Journal of Experimental Psychology*, 1964, *68*, 423–434.

Evans, S.H., & Anastasio, E.J. Misuse of analysis of covariance when treatment effect and covariate are confounded. *Psychological Bulletin*, 1968, *69*, 225–234.

Eysenck, M.W. Age differences in incidental learning. *Developmental Psychology*, 1974, *10*, 936–941.

Eysenck, M.W. Retrieval from semantic memory as a function of age. *Journal of Gerontology*, 1975, *30*, 174–180.

Falk, J.L., & Kline, D.W. Stimulus persistence and arousal. *Experimental Aging Research*, 1978, *4*, 109–123.

Farkas, M.S., & Hoyer, W.J. Processing consequences of perceptual grouping in selective attention. *Journal of Gerontology*, 1980, *35*, 207–216.

Farmer, A., McLean, S., Sparks, R., & O'Connell, P.F. Young adult, geriatric and aphasic group responses to simple analogies. *Journal of the American Geriatric Society*, 1978, *26*, 320–323.

Farquhar, M., & Leibowitz, H. The magnitude of the Ponzo illusion as a function of age for large and small configurations. *Psychonomic Science*, 1971, *25*, 97–98.

Farrimond, T. Visual and auditory performance variations with age: Some implications. *Australian Journal of Psychology*, 1967, *19*, 193–201.

Feier, C.D., & Gerstman, L.J. Sentence comprehension abilities throughout the adult life span. *Journal of Gerontology*, 1980, *35*, 722–728.

Ferree, C.E., Rand, G., & Monroe, M.M. A study of the factors which cause individual differences in the size of the form field. *American Journal of Psychology*, 1930, *42*, 63–71.

Ferris, S.H., Crook, T., Clark, E., McCarthy, M., & Rae, D. Facial recognition memory deficits in normal aging and senile dementia. *Journal of Gerontology*, 1980, *35*, 707–714.

Ford, J.M., Roth, W.T., Mohs, R.C., Hopkins, W.F., & Kopell, B.S. Event-related potentials recorded from young and old adults during a memory retrieval task. *Electroencephalography and Clinical Neurophysiology*, 1979, *47*, 450–459.

Fortuin, G.J. Age and lighting needs. *Ergonomics*, 1963, *6*, 239–245.

Foster, J.C., & Taylor, G.A. The application of mental tests to persons over 50. *Journal of Applied Psychology*, 1920, *4*, 29–58.

Foulds, G.A., & Raven, J.C. Normal changes in the mental abilities of adults as age advances. *Journal of Mental Science*, 1948, *94*, 133–142.

Fozard, J.L. Predicting age in the adult years from psychological assessments of abilities and personality. *Aging and Human Development*, 1972, *3*, 175–182.

Fozard, J.L., & Nuttall, R.L. General aptitude test battery scores for men differing in age and socioeconomic status. *Journal of Applied Psychology*, 1971, *55*, 372–379.

Fozard, J.L., & Popkin, S.J. Optimizing adult developmentnt: Ends and means of an applied psychology of aging. *American Psychologist*, 1978, *33*, 975–989.

Fozard, J.L., & Waugh, N.C. Proactive inhibition of prompted items. *Psychonomic Science*, 1969, *17*, 67–68.

Franklin, H.C., & Holding, D.H. Personal memories at different ages. *Quarterly Journal of Experimental Psychology*, 1977, *29*, 527–532.

Frederickson, W.A., & Geurin, J. Age differences in perceptual judgment on the Mueller-Lyer illusion. *Perceptual and Motor Skills*, 1973, *36*, 131–135.

Friedman, H. Memory organization in the aged. *Journal of Genetic Psychology*, 1966, *109*, 3–8.

Friedman, H. Interrelation of two types of immediate memory in the aged. *Journal of Psychology*, 1974, *87*, 177–181.

Friend, C.M., & Zubek, J.P. The effects of age on critical thinking ability. *Journal of Gerontology*, 1958, *13*, 407–413.

Fullerton, A.M. & Smith, A.D. Age-related differences in the use of redundancy. *Journal of Gerontology*, 1980, *35*, 729–735.

Furry, C.A., & Baltes, P.B. The effect of age differences in ability-extraneous performance variables on the assessment of intelligence in children, adults, and the elderly. *Journal of Gerontology*, 1973, *28*, 73–80.

Galton, F. On the anthropometric laboratory at the late International Health Exhibition. *Journal of the Anthropological Institute*, 1885, *14*, 205–218.

Ganzler, H. Motivation as a factor in the psychological deficit of aging. *Journal of Gerontology*, 1964, *19*, 425–429.

Gardner, E.F., & Monge, R.H. Adult age differences in cognitive abilities and educational background. *Experimental Aging Research*, 1977, *3*, 337–383.

Garfield, S.L., & Blek, L. Age, vocabulary level, and mental impairment. *Journal of Consulting Psychology*, 1952, *16*, 395–398.

Garrison, S.C. Retests on adults at an interval of ten years. *School and Society*, 1930, *32*, 326–328.

Gaylord, S.A., & Marsh, G.R. Age differences in the speed of a spatial cognitive process. *Journal of Gerontology*, 1976, *30*, 674–678.

Giambra, L.M., & Arenberg, D. Problem solving, concept learning, and aging. In L.W. Poon (Ed.), *Aging in the 1980's*. Washington, D.C.: American Psychological Association, 1980.

Gilbert, J.G. Memory efficiency in senescence. *Archives of Psychology*, 1935, *27* (Whole No. 188).

Gilbert, J.C. Memory loss in senescence. *Journal of Abnormal and Social Psychology*, 1941, *36*, 73–86.

Gilbert, J.C., & Levee, R.T. Patterns of declining memory. *Journal of Gerontology*, 1971, *26*, 70–75.

Girotti, G., & Beretta, A. Apparent verticality following short-term sensory deprivation: Differential performances in young and old men. *Cortex*, 1969, *5*, 74–86.

Gladis, M., & Braun, H.W. Age differences in transfer and retroaction as a function of intertask response similarity. *Journal of Experimental Psychology*, 1958, *55*, 25–30.

Glanzer, M., & Glaser, R. Cross-sectional and longitudinal results in a study of age-related changes. *Educational and Psychological Measurement*, 1959, *19*, 89–101.

Glanzer, M., Glaser, R., & Richlin, M. *Development of a test battery for study of age-related changes in intellectual and perceptual abilities*. Randolph A.F.B., Texas: USAF School of Aviation Medicine, 1958.

Goldfarb, W. *An Investigation of Reaction Time in Older Adults*. New York: Teachers College, Columbia University, 1941.

Gordon, S.K. Organization and recall of related sentences by elderly and young adults. *Experimental Aging Research*, 1975, *1*, 71–80.

Gordon, S.K., & Clark, W.C. Application of signal detection theory to prose recall and recognition in elderly and young adults. *Journal of Gerontology*, 1974, *29*, 64–72. (a)

Gordon, S.K., & Clark, W.C. Adult age differences in word and nonsense syllable recognition memory and response criterion. *Journal of Gerontology*, 1974, *29*, 659–665. (b)

Granick, S., & Friedman, A.D. The effect of education on the decline of psychometric test performance with age. *Journal of Gerontology*, 1967, *22*, 191–195.

Granick, S., Kleban, M.H., & Weiss, A.D. Relationships between hearing loss and cognition in normally hearing aged persons. *Journal of Gerontology*, 1976, *31*, 434–440.

Green, R.F. Age-intelligence relationship between ages sixteen and sixty-four: A rising trend. *Developmental Psychology*, 1969, *1*, 618–627.

Green, R.F., & Berkowitz, B. Changes in intellect with age: II. Factorial analysis of Wechsler-Bellevue scores. *Journal of Genetic Psychology*, 1964, *104*, 3–18.

Green, R.F., & Reimanis, G. The age-intelligence relationship—Longitudinal studies can mislead. *Industrial Gerontology*, 1970, *6*, 1–16.

Griew, S. A note on the effect of interrupting auditory signals on the performance of younger and older subjects. *Gerontologia*, 1958, *2*, 136–139.

Griew, S. Methodological problems in industrial ageing. *Occupational Psychology*, 1959, *33*, 36–46. (a)

Griew, S. Complexity of response and time of initiating responses in relation to age. *American Journal of Psychology*, 1959, *72*, 83–88. (b)

Griew, S. Age, information transmission, and the positional relationship between signals and responses in the performance of a choice task. *Ergonomics*, 1964, *7*, 267–277.

Griew, S., Fellows, B.J., & Howes, R. Duration of spiral aftereffect as a function of stimulus exposure and age. *Perceptual and Motor Skills*, 1963, *17*, 210.

Griew, S., & Tucker, W.A. The identification of job activities associated with age differences in the engineering industry. *Journal of Applied Psychology*, 1958, *42*, 278–282.

Guth, S.K. Effects of age on visibility. *American Journal of Optometry,* 1957, *34,* 463–477.

Guttman, R. Performance on the Raven Progessive Matrices as a function of age, education, and sex. *Educational Gerontology,* 1981, *7,* 49–55.

Haber, R.N., & Standing, L.G. Direct measures of short-term visual storage. *Quarterly Journal of Experimental Psychology,* 1969, *21,* 43–54.

Harkins, S.W., Chapman, C.R., & Eisdorfer, C. Memory loss and response bias in senescence. *Journal of Gerontology,* 1979, *34,* 66–72.

Hartley, A.A. Adult age differences in deductive reasoning processes. *Journal of Gerontology,* 1981, *36,* 700–706.

Hartley, J.T., Harker, J.O., & Walsh, D.A. Contemporary issues and new directions in adult development of learning and memory. In L.W. Poon (Ed.), *Aging in the 1980's.* Washington, D.C.: American Psychological Association, 1980.

Hartley, J.T., & Walsh, D.A. The effect of monetary incentive on amount and rate of free recall in older and younger adults. *Journal of Gerontology,* 1980, *35,* 899–905.

Harwood, E., & Naylor, G.F.K. Recall and recognition in elderly and young subjects. *Australian Journal of Psychology,* 1969, *21,* 251–257.

Hasher, L., & Zacks, R.T. Automatic and effortful processes in memory. *Journal of Experimental Psychology: General,* 1979, *108,* 356–388.

Hawkins, H.L., & Shulman, G.L. Two definitions of persistence in visual perception. *Perception and Psychophysics,* 1979, *25,* 348–350.

Hayslip, B., & Sterns, H.L. Age differences in relationships between crystallized and fluid intelligences and problem solving. *Journal of Gerontology,* 1979, *34,* 404–414.

Haywood, K.M. Coincidence-anticipation accuracy across the life span. *Experimental Aging Research,* 1980, *6,* 451–462.

Heglin, H.J. Problem solving set in different age groups. *Journal of Gerontology,* 1956, *11,* 310–317.

Helander, J. *On Age and Mental Test Behavior.* Goteborg, Sweden: Acta Psychologica Gothoburgensia, 1967.

Herman, J.F., & Coyne, A.C. Mental manipulation of spatial information in young and elderly adults. *Developmental Psychology,* 1980, *16,* 537–538.

Heron, A., & Chown, S.M. *Age and Function.* London: Churchill, 1967.

Heron, A., & Craik, F.I.M. Age differences in cumulative learning of meaningful and meaningless material. *Scandinavian Journal of Psychology,* 1964, *5,* 209–217.

Hertzog, C.K., Williams, M.V., & Walsh, D.A. The effects of practice on age differences in central perceptual processing. *Journal of Gerontology,* 1976, *31,* 428–433.

Heston, J.C., & Cannell, C.F. A note on the relation between age and performance of adult subjects on four familiar psychometric tests. *Journal of Applied Psychology,* 1941, *25,* 415–419.

Hills, B.L. Vision, visibility, and perception in driving. *Perception,* 1980, *9,* 183–216.

Hooper, F.H., & Sheehan, N.W. Logical concept attainment during the adult years. In W.F. Overton & J.M. Gallagher (Eds.), *Knowledge and Development* (Vol. 1). New York: Plenum Press, 1977.

Horn, J.L. Intelligence: Why it grows, why it declines. *Transaction,* 1967, *4,* 23–31.

Horn, J.L. Organization of data on life span development of human abilities. In L.R. Goulet & P.B. Baltes (Eds.), *Life Span Developmental Psychology: Research and Theory.* New York: Academic Press, 1970.

Horn, J.L. Psychometric studies of aging and intelligence. In S. Gershon & A. Raskin (Eds.), *Aging (Vol.2): Genesis and Treatment of Psychological Disorders in the Elderly.* New York: Raven Press, 1975.

Horn, J.L. Human ability systems. In P.B. Baltes (Ed.), *Life Span Development and Behavior* (Vol.1). New York: Academic Press, 1978.

Horn, J.L., & Cattell, R.B. Age differences in primary mental ability factors. *Journal of Gerontology,* 1966, *21,* 210–220.

Horn, J.L., & Cattell, R.B. Age differences in fluid and crystallized intelligence. *Acta Psychologica,* 1967, *26,* 107–129.

Horn, J.L., & Donaldson, G. On the myth of intellectual decline in adulthood. *American Psychologist,* 1976, *31,* 701–709.

Horn, J.L., & Donaldson, G. Faith is not enough: A response to the Baltes-Schaie claim that intelligence does not wane. *American Psychologist,* 1977, *32,* 369–373.

Horn, J.L., & Donaldson, G. Cognitive development in adulthood. In O.G. Brim & J. Kagan (Eds.), *Constancy and Change in Human Development.* Cambridge, Mass.: Harvard University Press, 1980.

Horn, J.L., Donaldson, G., & Engstrom, R. Apprehension, memory, and fluid intelligence decline in adulthood. *Research on Aging,* 1981, *3,* 33–84.

Howard, D. Category Norms: A comparison of the Battig and Montague (1969) Norms with the responses of adults between the ages of 20 and 80. *Journal of Gerontology,* 1980, *35,* 225–231.

Howard, D.V., Lasaga, M.I., & McAndrews, M.P. Semantic activation during memory encoding across the adult life span. *Journal of Gerontology,* 1980, *35,* 884–890.

Howard, D.V., McAndrews, M.P., & Lasaga, M.I. Semantic priming of lexical decisions in young and old adults. *Journal of Gerontology,* 1981, *36,* 707–714.

Howell, R.J. Sex differences and educational influences on a mental deterioration scale. *Journal of Gerontology,* 1955, *10,* 190–193.

Howell, S.C. Familiarity and complexity in perceptual recognition. *Journal of Gerontology,* 1972, *27,* 364–371.

Howes, D. Vocabulary size estimated from the distribution of word frequencies. In H. Mylebust (Ed.), *Progress in Learning Disabilities.* New York: Grune & Stratton, 1971.

Hoyer, W.J., Labouvie, G.V., & Baltes, P.B. Modification of response speed deficits and intellectual performance in the elderly. *Human Development,* 1973, *16,* 233–242.

Hoyer, W.J., Rebok, G.W., & Sved, S.M. Effects of varying irrelevant information on adult age differences in problem solving. *Journal of Gerontology,* 1979, *34,* 553–560.

Hulicka, I.M. Age differences for intentional and incidental learning and recall scores. *Journal of the American Geriatrics Society,* 1965, *13,* 639–649.

Hulicka, I.M. Age differences in Wechsler Memory Scale scores. *Journal of Genetic Psychology,* 1966, *109,* 135–146.

Hulicka, I.M. Age changes and age differences in memory functioning. *Gerontologist,* 1967, *7,* 46–54. (a)

Hulicka, I.M. Age differences in retention as a function of interference. *Journal of Gerontology,* 1967, *22,* 180–184. (b)

Hulicka, I.M., & Grossman, J.L. Age group comparisons for the use of mediators in paired-associate learning. *Journal of Gerontology,* 1967, *22,* 46–51.

Hulicka, I.M., & Rust, L.D. Age-related retention deficit as a function of learning. *Journal of the American Geriatrics Society,* 1964, *11,* 1061–1065.

Hulicka, I.M., Sterns, H., & Grossman, J. Age group comparisons of paired-associate learning as a function of paced and self-paced association and response times. *Journal of Gerontology*, 1967, *22*, 274–280.

Hulicka, I.M., & Weiss, R. Age differences in retention as a function of learning. *Journal of Consulting Psychology*, 1965, *29*, 125–129.

Hultsch, D.F. Adult age differences in the organization of free recall. *Developmental Psychology*, 1969, *1*, 673–678.

Hultsch, D.F. Organization and memory in adulthood. *Human Development*, 1971, *14*, 16–29. (a)

Hultsch, D.F. Adult age differences in free classification and free recall. *Developmental Psychology*, 1971, *4*, 338–342. (b)

Hultsch, D.F. Learning how to learn in adulthood. *Journal of Gerontology*, 1974, *29*, 302–308.

Hultsch, D.F. Adult age differences in retrieval: Trace-dependent and cue-dependent forgetting. *Developmental Psychology*, 1975, *11*, 197–201.

Huntington, J.M., & Simonson, E. Critical flicker fusion frequency as a function of exposure time in two different age groups. *Journal of Gerontology*, 1965, *20*, 527–529.

Inglis, J. & Ankus, M.N. Effects of age on short-term storage and serial rote learning. *British Journal of Psychology*, 1965, *56*, 183–195.

Inglis, J., Ankus, M.N., & Sykes, D.H. Age related differences in learning and short-term memory from childhood to senium. *Human Development*, 1968, *11*, 42–52.

Inglis, J., & Caird, W.K. Age differences in successive responses to simultaneous stimulation. *Canadian Journal of Psychology*, 1963, *17*, 98–105.

Inglis, J., & Tansey, C.L. Age differences and scoring differences in dichotic listening performance. *Journal of Psychology*, 1967, *66*, 325–332.

Jacewicz, M.M., & Hartley, A.A. Rotation of mental images by young and old college students: The effects of familiarity. *Journal of Gerontology*, 1979, *34*, 396–403.

Jani, S.H. The age factor in stereopses screening. *American Journal of Optometry*, 1966, *43*, 653–655.

Jaquish, G.A., & Ripple, R.E. Cognitive creative abilities and self-esteem across the adult life span. *Human Development*, 1981, *24*, 110–119.

Jenkins, J.J., & Russell, W.A. Systematic changes in word association norms: 1910–1952. *Journal of Abnormal and Social Psychology*, 1960, *60*, 293–304.

Jerome, E.A. Decay of heuristic processes in the aged. In C. Tibbitts & W. Donahue (Eds.), *Social and Psychological Aspects of Aging*. New York: Columbia University Press, 1962.

Johnson, M.K., & Raye, C.L. Reality monitoring. *Psychological Review*, 1981, *88*, 67–85.

Jones, H.E. Age changes in mental abilities. In *Old Age and the Modern World*. Edinburgh: Livingstone, 1955.

Jones, H.E. Problems of aging in perceptual and intellective functions. In J.E. Anderson (Ed.), *Psychological Aspects of Aging*. Washington, D.C.: American Psychological Association, 1956.

Jones, H.E. Intelligence and problem solving. In J.E. Birren (Ed.), *Handbook of the Aging and the Individual*. Chicago: University of Chicago Press, 1959.

Jones, H.E., & Conrad, H.S. The growth and decline of intelligence: A study of a homogeneous group between the ages of ten and sixty. *Genetic Psychology Monographs*, 1933, *13*, 223–298.

Jones, H.E., Conrad, H.S., & Horn, A. Psychological studies of motion pictures: II. Observation and recall as a function of age. *University of California Publications in Psychology*, 1928, *3*, 225–243.

Jones, H.E., & Kaplan, O.J. Psychological aspects of mental disorders in later life. In O.J. Kaplan (Ed.), *Mental Disorders in Later Life*. Stanford, Calif.: Stanford University Press, 1945.

Kahneman, D. *Attention and Effort*. Englewood Cliffs, N.J.: Prentice-Hall, 1973.

Kamin, L.J. Differential changes in mental abilities in old age. *Journal of Gerontology*, 1957, *12*, 66–70.

Kangas, J. & Bradway, K. Intelligence at middle age: A thirty-eight-year follow-up. *Developmental Psychology*, 1971, *5*, 333–337.

Kantowitz, B.H. Double stimulation. In B.H. Kantowitz (Ed.), *Human Information Processing: Tutorials in Performance and Cognition*. Hillsdale, N.J.: Lawrence Erlbaum Associates, 1974.

Kaplan, O.J. The place of psychology in gerontology. *Geriatrics*, 1951, *6*, 298–303.

Kastenbaum, R.J. & Candy, S.E. The 4% fallacy: A methodological and empirical critique of extended care facility population statistics. *International Journal of Aging*, 1973, *4*, 15–21.

Kausler, D.H. Imagery ratings for young and elderly adults. *Experimental Aging Research*, 1980, *6*, 185–188.

Kausler, D.H., Hakami, M.K., & Wright, R.E. Adult age differences in frequency judgments of categorical representation. *Journal of Gerontology*, 1982, *37*, 365–371.

Kausler, D.H., & Kleim, D.M. Age differences in processing relevant versus irrelevant stimuli in multiple-item recognition learning. *Journal of Gerontology*, 1978, *33*, 87–93.

Kausler, D.H., Kleim, D.M., & Overcast, T.D. Item recognition following a multiple-item study trial for young and middle-aged adults. *Experimental Aging Research*, 1975, *2*, 243–250.

Kausler, D.H., & Lair, C.J. R-S (backward) paired-associate learning in elderly subjects. *Journal of Gerontology*, 1965, *20*, 29–31.

Kausler, D.H., & Lair, C.J. Associative strength and paired-associate learning in elderly subjects. *Journal of Gerontology*, 1966, *21*, 278–280.

Kausler, D.H., & Puckett, J.M. Effects of word frequency on adult age differences in word memory span. *Experimental Aging Research*, 1979, *5*, 161–169.

Kausler, D.H., & Puckett, J.M. Frequency judgments and correlated cognitive abilities in young and elderly adults. *Journal of Gerontology*, 1980, *35*, 376–382. (a)

Kausler, D.H., & Puckett, J.M. Adult age differences in recognition memory for a non-semantic attribute. *Experimental Aging Research*, 1980, *6*, 349–356. (b)

Kausler, D.H., & Puckett, J.M. Adult age differences in memory for sex of voice. *Journal of Gerontology*, 1981, *36*, 44–50. (a)

Kausler, D.H., & Puckett, J.M. Adult age differences in memory for modality attributes. *Experimental Aging Research*, 1981, *7*, 117–125. (b)

Kausler, D.H., Wright, R.E. & Hakami, M.K. Variation in task complexity and adult age differences in frequency-of-occurrence judgments. *Bulletin of the Psychonomic Society*, 1981, *18*, 195–197.

Kear-Calwell, J.J., & Heller, M. A normative study of the Wechsler Memory Scale. *Journal of Clinical Psychology*, 1978, *34*, 437–442.

Keevil-Rogers, P., & Schnore, M.M. Short-term memory as a function of age in persons of above average intelligence. *Journal of Gerontology*, 1969, *24*, 184–188.

Kendall, B.S. Memory for Designs performance in the seventh and eighth decades of life. *Perceptual and Motor Skills,* 1962, *14,* 399–405.

Kennedy, K.J. Age effects on Trail-Making Test performance. *Perceptual and Motor Skills,* 1981, *52,* 671–675.

Kesler, M.S., Denney, N.W., & Whitely, S.E. Factors influencing problem solving in middle-aged and elderly adults. *Human Development,* 1976, *19,* 310–320.

King, H.F. An attempt to use production data in the study of age and performance. *Journal of Gerontology,* 1956, *11,* 410–416.

Kinsbourne, M. Age effects on letter span related to rate and sequential dependency. *Journal of Gerontology,* 1973, *28,* 317–319.

Kinsbourne, M. Cognitive deficit and the aging brain: A behavioral analysis. *International Journal of Aging and Human Development,* 1974, *5,* 41–49.

Kinsbourne, M., & Berryhill, J.L. The nature of the interaction between pacing and the age decrement in learning. *Journal of Gerontology,* 1972, *27,* 471–477.

Kirchner, W.K. Age differences in short-term retention of rapidly changing information. *Journal of Experimental Psychology,* 1958, *55,* 352–358.

Kline, D.W., & Baffa, G. Differences in the sequential integration of form as a function of age and interstimulus interval. *Experimental Aging Research,* 1976, *2,* 333–343.

Kline, D.W., & Birren, J.E. Age differences in backward dichoptic masking. *Experimental Aging Research,* 1975, *1,* 17–25.

Kline, D.W., Culler, M.P., & Sucec, J. Differences in inconspicuous word identification as a function of age and reversible-figure training. *Experimental Aging Research,* 1977, *3,* 203–213.

Kline, D.W., Hogan, P.M., & Stier, D.L. Age and the identification of inconspicuous words. *Experimental Aging Research,* 1980, *6,* 137–147.

Kline, D.W., & Nestor, S. Persistence of complementary afterimages as a function of adult age and exposure duration. *Experimental Aging Research,* 1977, *3,* 191–201.

Kline, D.W., & Orme-Rogers, C. Examination of stimulus persistence as the basis for superior visual identification performance among older adults. *Journal of Gerontology,* 1978, *33,* 76–81.

Kline, D.W., & Scheiber, F. What are the age differences in visual sensory memory? *Journal of Gerontology,* 1981, *36,* 86–89. (a)

Kline, D.W., & Scheiber, F. Visual aging: A transient/sustained shift? *Perception and Psychophysics,* 1981, *29,* 181–182. (b)

Kline, D.W., & Szafran, J. Age differences in backward monoptic visual noise masking. *Journal of Gerontology,* 1975, *30,* 307–311.

Klodin, V.M. The relationship of scoring treatment and age in perceptual-integrative performance. *Experimental Aging Research,* 1976, *2,* 303–313.

Kogan, N. Categorizing and conceptualizing styles in younger and older adults. *Human Development,* 1974, *17,* 218–230.

Kohn, M.L., & Schooler, C. The reciprocal effects of the substantive complexity of work and intellectual flexibility: A longitudinal assessment. *American Journal of Sociology,* 1978, *84,* 24–52.

Korchin, S.J., & Basowitz, H. Age differences in verbal learning. *Journal of Abnormal and Social Psychology,* 1957, *54,* 64–69.

Kriauciunas, R. The relationship of age and retention interval activity in short-term memory. *Journal of Gerontology,* 1968, *23,* 169–173.

Kuhlen, R.G. Social change: A neglected factor in psychological studies of the life span. *School and Society,* 1940, *52,* 14–16.

Kuhlen, R.G. Age and intelligence: The significance of cultural change in longitudinal vs. cross-sectional findings. *Vita Humana*, 1963, *6*, 113–124.

Kutscher, R.E., & Walker, J.F. Comparative job performance of office workers by age. *Monthly Labor Review*, 1960, *83*, 39–43.

Lachman, J.L., Lachman, R. & Thronesberry, C. Metamemory through the adult life span. *Developmental Psychology*, 1979, *15*, 543–551.

Lair, C.J., Moon, W.H., & Kausler, D.H. Associative interference in the paired-associate learning of middle-aged and old subjects. *Developmental Psychology*, 1969, *9*, 548–552.

Langer, E.J., Rodin, J., Beck, P., Weinman, C., & Spitzer, L. Environmental determinants of memory improvement in late adulthood. *Journal of Personality and Social Psychology*, 1979, *37*, 2003–2013.

Laurence, M.W. Age differences in performance and subjective organization in the free-recall learning of pictorial material. *Canadian Journal of Psychology*, 1966, *20*, 388–399.

Laurence, M.W. Memory loss with age: A test of two strategies for its retardation. *Psychonomic Science*, 1967, *9*, 209–210.

Laurence, M.W., & Trotter, M. Effect of acoustic factors and list organization in multi-trial free-recall learning of college-age and elderly adults. *Developmental Psychology*, 1971, *5*, 202–210.

Layton, B. Perceptual noise and aging. *Psychological Bulletin*, 1975, *82*, 875–883.

Lee, J.A., & Pollack, R.A. The effects of age on perceptual problem-solving strategies. *Experimental Aging Research*, 1978, *4*, 37–54.

Lefever, D.W., Van Boven, A., & Banarer, J. Relation of test scores to age and education for adult workers. *Educational and Psychological Measurement*, 1946, *6*, 351–360.

Lehman, H.C. *Age and Achievement*. Princeton, N.J.: Princeton University Press, 1953.

Lehman, H.C. Man's creative production rate at different ages and in different countries. *Scientific Monthly*, 1954, *78*, 321–326.

Lehman, H.C. The chemist's most creative years. *Science*, 1958, *127*, 1213–1222. (a)

Lehman, H.C. The influence of longevity upon curves showing man's creative production rate at successive age levels. *Journal of Gerontology*, 1958, *13*, 187–191. (b)

Lehman, H.C. The creative production rates of present versus past generations of scientists. *Journal of Gerontology*, 1962, *17*, 409–417.

Leibowitz, H.W., & Judisch, J.M. The relation between age and the magnitude of the Ponzo Illusion. *American Journal of Psychology*, 1967, *80*, 105–109.

Lienert, G.A., & Crott, H.W. Studies on the factor structure of intelligence in children, adolescents, and adults. *Vita Humana*, 1964, *7*, 147–163.

Looft, W.R. Note on WAIS Vocabulary performance by young and old adults. *Psychological Reports*, 1970, *26*, 943–946.

Lorden, R., Atkeson, B.M., & Pollack, R.H. Differences in the magnitude of the Delboeuf illusion and Usnadze effect during adulthood. *Journal of Gerontology*, 1979, *34*, 229–233.

Lorge, I. Methodology of the study of intelligence and emotion in ageing. In G.E.W. Wolstenholme & C.M. O'Connor (Eds.), *Ciba Foundation Colloquia on Ageing*. Boston, Mass.: Little, Brown and Co., 1957.

Ludwig, T.E. Age differences in mental synthesis. *Journal of Gerontology*, 1982, *37*, 182–189.

Mackay, H.A., & Inglis, J. The effects of age on short-term auditory storage processes. *Gerontologia*, 1963, *8*, 193–200.

Madden, D.J., & Nebes, R.D. Aging and the development of automaticity in visual search. *Developmental Psychology*, 1980, *16*, 377–384.

Maher, H. Age and performance of two work groups. *Journal of Gerontology*, 1955, *10*, 448–451.

Manniche, E., & Falk, G. Age and the Nobel Prize. *Behavioral Science*, 1957, *2*, 301–307.

Mark, J.A. Measurement of job performance and age. *Monthly Labor Review*, 1956, *79*, 1410–1414.

Mark, J.A. Comparative job performance by age. *Monthly Labor Review*, 1957, *80*, 1467–1471.

Marsh, B.W. Aging and driving. *Traffic Engineering*, 1960 (November), 3–21.

Marsh, G.A. Age differences in evoked potential correlates of a memory-scanning process. *Experimental Aging Research*, 1975, *1*, 3–16.

Marshall, P.H., Elias, J.W., Webber, S.M., Gist, B.A., Winn, F.J., & King, P. Age differences in verbal mediation: A structural and functional analysis. *Experimental Aging Research*, 1978, *4*, 175–193.

Mason, C.F., & Ganzler, H. Adult norms for the Shipley Institute of Living Scale and Hooper Visual Organization Test based on age and education. *Journal of Gerontology*, 1964, *19*, 419–424.

Mason, S.E. Effects of orienting tasks on the recall and recognition performance of subjects differing in age. *Developmental Psychology*, 1979, *15*, 467–469.

Mason, S.E., & Smith, A.D. Imagery in the aged. *Experimental Aging Research*, 1977, *3*, 17–32.

Maule, A.J., & Sanford, A.J. Adult age differences in multi-source selection behavior with partially predictable signals. *British Journal of Psychology*, 1980, *71*, 69–81.

McCormack, P.D. Autobiographical memory in the aged. *Canadian Journal of Psychology*, 1979, *33*, 118–124.

McCormack, P.D. Temporal coding by young and elderly adults: A test of the Hasher-Zacks model. *Developmental Psychology*, 1981, *17*, 509–515.

McCormack, P.D. Coding of spatial information by young and elderly adults. *Journal of Gerontology*, 1982, *37*, 80–86.

McFarland, R.A. *Human Factors in Air Transportation and Occupational Health and Safety*. New York: McGraw-Hill, 1953.

McFarland, R.A. The need for functional age measurements in industrial gerontology. *Industrial Gerontology*, 1973, *19*, 1–19.

McFarland, R.A., Domey, R.G., Warren, A.B., & Ward, D.C. Dark adaptation as a function of age: I. A statistical analysis. *Journal of Gerontology*, 1960, *15*, 149–154.

McFarland, R.A., & Fisher, M.B. Alterations in dark adaptation as a function of age. *Journal of Gerontology*, 1955, *10*, 424–428.

McFarland, R.A., Moseley, A.L., & Fisher, M.B. Age and the problems of professional truck drivers in highway transportation. *Journal of Gerontology*, 1954, *9*, 338–348.

McFarland, R.A., & O'Doherty, B.M. Work and occupational skills. In J.E. Birren (Ed.), *Handbook of Aging and the Individual*. Chicago: University of Chicago Press, 1959.

McFarland, R.A., Tune, C.S., & Welford, A.T. On the driving of automobiles by older people. *Journal of Gerontology*, 1964, *19*, 190–197.

McFarland, R.A., Warren, A.B., & Karis, C. Alterations in critical flicker frequency as a function of age and light-dark interval. *Journal of Experimental Psychology*, 1958, *56*, 529–538.

McGee, M.G. Human spatial abilities: Psychometric studies and environmental, genetic, hormonal, and neurological influences. *Psychological Bulletin*, 1979, *86*, 889–918.

McGhie, A., Chapman, J., & Lawson, J.S. Changes in immediate memory with age. *British Journal of Psychology*, 1965, *56*, 69–75.

McHugh, R.B., & Owens, W.A. Age changes in mental organization: A longitudinal study. *Journal of Gerontology*, 1954, *9*, 296–302.

McNulty, J.A., & Caird, W.K. Memory loss with age: Retrieval or storage. *Psychological Reports*, 1966, *19*, 229–230.

Mergler, N.L., Dusek, J.B., & Hoyer, W.J. Central/incidental recall and selective attention in young and elderly adults. *Experimental Aging Research*, 1977, *3*, 49–60.

Mergler, N.L., & Hoyer, W.J. Effects of training on dimensional classification abilities: Adult age comparisons. *Educational Gerontology*, 1981, *6*, 135–145.

Meyer, B.J., & Rice, G.E. Information recalled from prose by young, middle, and old adult readers. *Experimental Aging Research*, 1981, *7*, 253–268.

Miles, C.C. Influence of speed and age on intelligence scores of adults. *Journal of Genetic Psychology*, 1934, *10*, 208–210.

Miles, C.C., & Miles, W.R. The correlation of intelligence scores and chronological age from early to late maturity. *American Journal of Psychology*, 1932, *44*, 44–78.

Miles, W.R. Age and human ability. *Psychological Review*, 1933, *40*, 99–123.

Miles, W.R. Training, practice, and mental longevity. *Science*, 1935, *81*, 79–87.

Misiak, H. Age and sex differences in critical flicker frequency. *Journal of Experimental Psychology*, 1947, *37*, 318–332.

Misiak, H. The decrease of critical flicker frequency with age. *Science*, 1951, *113*, 551–552.

Mistler-Lachman, J.L. Spontaneous shift in encoding dimensions among elderly subjects. *Journal of Gerontology*, 1977, *32*, 68–72.

Moenster, P.A. Learning and memory in relation to age. *Journal of Gerontology*, 1972, *27*, 361–363.

Monge, R.H. Studies of verbal learning from the college years through middle age. *Journal of Gerontology*, 1971, *26*, 324–329.

Monge, R.H., & Hultsch, D.F. Paired-associate learning as a function of adult age and the length of the anticipation and inspection intervals. *Journal of Gerontology*, 1971, *26*, 157–162.

Moray, N. Where is capacity limited? A survey and a model. In A.F. Sanders (Ed.), *Attention and Performance I*. Amsterdam: North-Holland, 1967.

Mueller, J.H., Kausler, D.H., Faherty, A., & Oliveri, M. Reaction time as a function of age, anxiety, and typicality. *Bulletin of the Psychonomic Society*, 1980, *16*, 473–476.

Muhs, P.J., Hooper, F.H., & Papalia-Finlay, D. Cross-sectional analysis of cognitive functioning across the life span. *International Journal of Aging and Human Development*, 1979, *10*, 311–333.

Murphy, M.D., Sanders, R.E., Gabriesheski, A.S., & Schmitt, F.A. Metamemory in the aged. *Journal of Gerontology*, 1981, *36*, 185–193.

Murrell, K.F.H. Industrial aspects of ageing. *Ergonomics*, 1962, *5*, 147–154.

Murrell, K.F.H. *Human Performance in Industry*. New York: Reinhold, 1965.

Murrell, K.F.H., & Edwards, E. Field studies of an indicator machine tool travel with special reference to the ageing worker. *Occupational Psychology,* 1963, *37,* 267–275.

Murrell, K.F.H., & Forsaith, B. Age and the timing of movement. *Occupational Psychology,* 1960, *34,* 275–279.

Murrell, K.F.H., & Griew, S. Age structure in the engineering industry: A study of regional effects. *Occupational Psychology,* 1958, *34,* 86–88.

Murrell, K.F.H., Griew, S., & Tucker, W.A. Age structure in the engineering industry: A preliminary study. *Occupational Psychology,* 1957, *31,* 150–168.

Murrell, K.F.H., & Humphries, S. Age, experience, and short-term memory. In M.M. Gruneberg, P.E. Morris, & R.N. Sykes (Eds.), *Practical Aspects of Memory.* London: Academic Press, 1978.

Murrell, K.F.H., Powesland, P.F. & Forsaith, B. A study of pillar-drilling in relation to age. *Occupational Psychology,* 1962, *36,* 45–52.

Murrell, K.F.H., & Tucker, M.A. A pilot job-study of age-related causes of difficulty in light engineering. *Ergonomics,* 1960, *3,* 74–79.

Mursell, G.R. Decrease in intelligence with increase in age among inmates of penal institutions. *Journal of Juvenile Research,* 1929, *13,* 199–203.

Nebes, R.D. Verbal-pictorial recoding in the elderly. *Journal of Gerontology,* 1976, *31,* 421–427.

Nebes, R.D., & Andrews-Kulis, M.E. The effect of age on the speed of sentence formation and incidental learning. *Experimental Aging Research,* 1976, *2,* 315–332.

Nehrke, M.F. Age, sex, and educational differences in syllogistic reasoning. *Journal of Gerontology,* 1972, *27,* 466–470.

Nehrke, M.F. Age and sex differences in discrimination learning and transfer of training. *Journal of Gerontology,* 1973, *28,* 320–327.

Neisser, U. *Cognition and Reality.* San Francisco, Calif.: Freeman, 1976.

Nickerson, R.S. Retrieval efficiency, knowledge assessment, and age: Comments on some welcome findings. In L.W. Poon, J.L. Fozard, L.S. Cermak, D. Arenberg, & L.W. Thompson (Eds.), *New Directions in Memory and Aging.* Hillsdale, N.J.: Lawrence Erlbaum Associates, 1980.

Nisbet, J.D. Intelligence and age: Retesting with twenty-four years' interval. *British Journal of Educational Psychology,* 1957, *27,* 190–198.

Norman, D.A., & Bobrow, D.G. On data-limited and resource-limited processes. *Cognitive Psychology,* 1975, *7,* 44–64.

Nuttall, R.L. The strategy of functional age research. *Aging and Human Development,* 1972, *3,* 149–152.

Offenbach, S.I. A developmental study of hypothesis testing and cue selection strategies. *Developmental Psychology,* 1974, *10,* 484–490.

Ohta, R.J., Walsh, D.A., & Krauss, I.K. Spatial perspective-taking ability in young and elderly adults. *Experimental Aging Research,* 1981, *7,* 45–63.

Okun, M.A. Adult age and cautiousness in decision: A review of the literature. *Human Development,* 1976, *19,* 220–223.

Okun, M.A., & DiVesta, F.J. Cautiousness in adulthood as a function of age and instructions. *Journal of Gerontology,* 1976, *31,* 571–576.

Okun, M.A., & Elias, C.S. Cautiousness in adulthood as a function of age and payoff structure. *Journal of Gerontology,* 1977, *32,* 451–455.

Okun, M.A., & Siegler, I.C. Relation between preference for intermediate risk and adult age in men: A cross-cultural validation. *Developmental Psychology,* 1976, *12,* 565–566.

Overall, J.E., & Gorham, D.R. Organicity versus old age in objective and projective test performance. *Journal of Consulting and Clinical Psychology,* 1972, *39,* 98–105.

Owens, W.A. Age and mental abilities: A longitudinal study. *Genetic Psychology Monographs,* 1953, *48,* 3–54.

Owens, W.A. Age and mental abilities: A second adult follow-up. *Journal of Educational Psychology,* 1966, *57,* 311–325.

Panek, P.E., Barrett, G.V., Sterns, H.L., & Alexander, R.A. Age differences in perceptual style, selective attention, and perceptual-motor reaction time. *Experimental Aging Research,* 1978, *4,* 377–387.

Panek, P.E., & Stoner, S.B. Age differences on Raven's Colored Progressive Matrices. *Perceptual and Motor Skills,* 1980, *50,* 977–978.

Papalia, D.E., & Bielby, D.D.V. Cognitive functioning in middle and old age adults: A review of research based on Piaget's theory. *Human Development,* 1974, *17,* 424–443.

Park, D.C., Puglisi, J.T., & Lutz, R. Spatial memory in older adults: Effects of intentionality. *Journal of Gerontology,* 1982, *37,* 330–335.

Parkinson, S.R., Lindholm, J.M., & Urell, T. Aging, dichotic memory, and digit span. *Journal of Gerontology,* 1980, *35,* 87–95.

Peak, D.T. Changes in short-term memory in a group of aging community residents. *Journal of Gerontology,* 1968, *23,* 9–16.

Pelz, D.C., & Andrews, F.M. *Scientists in Organizations.* New York: John Wiley and Sons, 1966.

Perlmutter, M. What is memory aging the aging of? *Developmental Psychology,* 1978, *14,* 330–345.

Perlmutter, M. Age differences in adult's free recall, cued recall, and recognition. *Journal of Gerontology,* 1979, *34,* 533–539. (a)

Perlmutter, M. Age differences in the consistency of adults' associative responses. *Experimental Aging Research,* 1979, *5,* 549–553. (b)

Perlmutter, M., Metzger, R., Miller, K., & Nezworski, T. Memory of historical events. *Experimental Aging Research,* 1980, *6,* 47–60.

Perlmutter, M., Metzger, R., Nezworski, T., & Miller, K. Spatial and temporal memory in 20 and 60 year olds. *Journal of Gerontology,* 1981, *36,* 59–65.

Phillips, L.W., & Sternthal, B. Age differences in information processing: A perspective on the aged consumer. *Journal of Marketing Research,* 1977, *14,* 444–457.

Planek, T.W. Factors influencing the adaptation of the aging driver to today's traffic. *Clinical Medicine,* 1974 (May), 36–43.

Planek, T.W., & Fowler, R.C. Traffic accident problems and exposure characteristics of the aging driver. *Journal of Gerontology,* 1971, *26,* 224–230.

Plemons, J.K., Willis, S.L., & Baltes, P.B. Modifiability of fluid intelligence in aging: A short-term longitudinal training approach. *Journal of Gerontology,* 1978, *33,* 224–231.

Plude, D.J., & Hoyer, W.J. Adult age differences in visual search as a function of stimulus mapping and processing load. *Journal of Gerontology,* 1981, *36,* 598–604.

Pollack, R.H. A theoretical note on the aging of the visual system. *Perception and Psychophysics,* 1978, *23,* 94–95.

Pollack, R.H. & Atkeson, B.M. A life-span approach to perceptual development. In P.B. Baltes (Ed.), *Life-Span Development and Behavior.* (Vol. 1). New York: Academic Press, 1978.

Poon, L.W., & Fozard, J.L. Speed of retrieval from long-term memory in relation to age, familiarity, and datedness of information. *Journal of Gerontology*, 1978, *33*, 711–717.

Poon, L.W., & Fozard, J.L. Age and word frequency effects in continuous recognition memory. *Journal of Gerontology*, 1980, *35*, 77–86.

Poon, L.W., Fozard, J.L., Paulshock, D.R., & Thomas, J.C. A questionnaire assessment of age differences in retention of recent and remote events. *Experimental Aging Research*, 1979, *5*, 401–411.

Poon, L.W., & Walsh-Sweeney, L. Effects of bizarre and interacting imagery on learning and retrieval of the aged. *Experimental Aging Research*, 1981, *7*, 65–70.

Price, B. The grasping of spoken directions as an age function in adults. *Psychological Bulletin*, 1933, *30*, 588–589.

Puglisi, J.T. Semantic encoding in older adults as evidenced by release from proactive inhibition. *Journal of Gerontology*, 1980, *35*, 743–745.

Rabbitt, P.M.A. An age decrement in the ability to ignore irrelevant information. *Journal of Gerontology*, 1965, *20*, 233–238. (a)

Rabbitt, P.M.A. Age and discrimination between complex stimuli. In A.T. Welford & J.E. Birren (Eds.), *Behavior, Aging and the Nervous System.* Springfield, Ill.: Charles C Thomas, 1965. (b)

Rabbitt, P.M.A. Changes in problem-solving ability in old age. In J.E. Birren & K.W. Schaie (Eds.), *Handbook of the Psychology of Aging.* New York: Van Nostrand Reinhold, 1977.

Radcliffe, J.A. WAIS factorial structure and factor scores for ages 18 to 54. *Australian Journal of Psychology*, 1966, *18*, 228–238.

Rajalakshmi, R., & Jeeves, M.A. Changes in tachistoscopic form perception as a function of age and intellectual status. *Journal of Gerontology*, 1963, *18*, 275–278.

Rankin, J.L. & Kausler, D.H. Adult age differences in false recognitions. *Journal of Gerontology*, 1979, *34*, 58–65.

Raven, J.C. The comparative assessment of intellectual ability. *British Journal of Psychology*, 1948, *39*, 12–19.

Raymond, B.J. Free recall among the aged. *Psychological Reports*, 1971, *29*, 1179–1182.

Reading, V.M. Visual resolution as measured by dynamic and static tests. *Pflugers Archiv*, 1972, *333*, 17–26.

Rebok, G.W. Age effects in problem solving in relation to irrelevant information, dimensional preferences, and feedback. *Experimental Aging Research*, 1981, *7*, 393–403.

Reed, H.B.C., & Reitan, R.M. Changes in psychological test performance associated with the normal aging process. *Journal of Gerontology*, 1963, *18*, 271–274.

Richards, O.W. Effects of luminance and contrast on visual acuity, ages 16 to 90 years. *American Journal of Optometry and Physiological Optics*, 1977, *54*, 178–184.

Riege, W.H., & Inman, V. Age differences in nonverbal memory tasks. *Journal of Gerontology*, 1981, *36*, 51–58.

Riege, W.H., Kelly, K., & Klane, L.T. Age and error differences on Memory for Designs. *Perceptual and Motor Skills*, 1981, *52*, 507–513.

Riegel, K.F. A study of verbal achievements of older persons. *Journal of Gerontology*, 1959, *14*, 453–456.

Riegel, K.F. Age and cultural differences as determinants of word associations: Suggestions for their analyses. *Psychological Reports*, 1965, *16*, 75–78.

Riegel, K.F., & Birren, J.E. Age differences in associative behavior. *Journal of Gerontology*, 1965, *20*, 125–130.

Riegel, K.F., & Riegel. R.M. Changes in associative behavior during later years of life: A cross-sectional analysis. *Vita Humana*, 1964, *7*, 1–32.

Riegel, K.F., & Riegel, R.M. Development, drop, and death. *Developmental Psychology*, 1972, *6*, 306–319.

Riegel, R.M., & Riegel, K.F. A comparison and reinterpretation of factorial structures of the W-B, the WAIS and the HAWIE on aged persons. *Journal of Consulting Psychology*, 1962, *26*, 31–37.

Robertson, G.W., & Yudkin, J. Effect of age upon dark adaptation. *Journal of Physiology*, 1944, *103*, 1–8.

Robertson-Tchabo, E.A., & Arenberg, D. Age differences in cognition in healthy educated men: A factor analysis of experimental measures. *Experimental Aging Research*, 1976, *2*, 75–89.

Ross, E. Effects of challenging and supportive instructions on verbal learning in older persons. *Journal of Educational Psychology*, 1968, *59*, 261–266.

Rowe, E.J. & Schnore, M.M. Item concreteness and reported strategies in paired-associate learning as a function of age. *Journal of Gerontology*, 1971, *24*, 470–475.

Ruch, F.L. The differentiative effects of age upon human learning. *Journal of General Psychology*, 1934, *11*, 261–285.

Salthouse, T.A. Age and tachistoscopic perception. *Experimental Aging Research*, 1976, *2*, 91–103.

Salthouse, T.A. Adult age and the speed-accuracy tradeoff. *Ergonomics*, 1979, *22*, 811–821.

Salthouse, T.A. Age and memory: Strategies for localizing the loss. In L.W. Poon, J.L. Fozard, L.S. Cermak, D. Arenberg, & L.W. Thompson (Eds.), *New Directions in Memory and Aging*. Hillsdale, N.J.: Lawrence Erlbaum Associates, 1980.

Salthouse, T.A. Motor performance and speed of behavior. In J.E. Birren & K.W. Schaie (Eds.), *Handbook of the Psychology of Aging*. New York: Van Nostrand Reinhold, in press.

Salthouse, T.A. & Kail, R. Memory development throughout the life span: The role of processing rate. In P.B. Baltes & O.G. Brim (Eds.), *Life Span Development and Behavior* (Vol. 5). New York: Academic Press, in press.

Salthouse, T.A., & Somberg, B.L. Isolating the age deficit in speeded performance. *Journal of Gerontology*, 1982, *37*, 59–63. (a)

Salthouse, T.A., & Somberg, B.L. Time-accuracy relationships in young and old adults. *Journal of Gerontology*, 1982, *37*, 349–357. (b)

Salthouse, T.A., & Somberg, B.L. Skilled performance: The effects of adult age and experience on elementary processes. *Journal of Experimental Psychology: General*, 1982, *111*, 176–207. (c)

Sanders, R.E., Murphy, M.D., Schmitt, F.A., & Walsh, K.K. Age differences in free-recall rehearsal strategies. *Journal of Gerontology*, 1980, *35*, 550–558.

Sanford, A.J. Age-related differences in strategies for locating hidden targets. *Gerontologia*, 1973, *19*, 16–21.

Sanford, A.J., & Maule, A.J. The allocation of attention in multi-source monitoring behavior: Adult age differences. *Perception*, 1973, *2*, 91–100.

Schaie, K.W. Rigidity-flexibility and intelligence: A cross-sectional study of the adult life span from 20 to 70. *Psychological Monographs*, 1958, *72* (462, Whole No. 9).

Schaie, K.W. A general model for the study of developmental problems. *Psychological Bulletin*, 1965, *64*, 92–107.

Schaie, K.W. Age changes and age differences. *Gerontologist*, 1967, *6*, 128–132.

Schaie, K.W. Limitations on the generalizability of growth curves on intelligence. *Human Development*, 1972, *15*, 141–152.

Schaie, K.W. Translations in gerontology—From lab to life: Intellectual functioning. *American Psychologist*, 1974, *29*, 802–807.

Schaie, K.W. Quasi-experimental research designs. In J.E. Birren & K.W. Schaie (Eds.), *Handbook of the Psychology of Aging*. New York: Van Nostrand Reinhold, 1977.

Schaie, K.W., & Baltes, P.B. On sequential strategies in developmental research and the Schaie-Baltes controversy: Description or explanation? *Human Development*, 1975, *18*, 384–390.

Schaie, K.W., & Labouvie-Vief, G. Generational versus ontogenetic components of change in adult cognitive behavior: A fourteen-year cross-sequential study. *Developmental Psychology*, 1974, *10*, 305–320.

Schaie, K.W., Labouvie, G.V., & Buech, B.V. Generational and cohort-specific differences in adult cognitive functioning: A fourteen-year study of independent samples. *Developmental Psychology*, 1973, *9*, 151–166.

Schaie, K.W., & Parham, I.A. Cohort-sequential analyses of adult intellectual development. *Developmental Psychology*, 1977, *13*, 649–653.

Schaie, K.W., Rosenthal, F., & Perlman, R.M. Differential mental deterioration of factorially "pure" functions in later maturity. *Journal of Gerontology*, 1953, *8*, 191–196.

Schaie, K.W., & Strother, C.R. A cross-sequential study of age changes in cognitive behavior. *Psychological Bulletin*, 1968, *70*, 671–680. (a)

Schaie, K.W., & Strother, C.R. The effects of time and cohort differences on the interpretation of age changes in cognitive behavior. *Multivariate Behavioral Research*, 1968, *3*, 259–294. (b)

Schear, J.M., & Nebes, R.D. Memory for verbal and spatial information as a function of age. *Experimental Aging Research*, 1980, *6*, 271–282.

Schmitt, F.A., Murphy, M.D., & Sanders, R.E. Training older adult free-recall rehearsal strategies. *Journal of Gerontology*, 1981, *36*, 329–337.

Schneider, N.G., Gritz, E.R., & Jarvik, M.E. Age differences in learning, immediate and one-week delayed recall. *Gerontolgia*, 1975, *21*, 10–20.

Schonfield, D. Memory changes with age. *Nature*, 1965, *208*, 918.

Schonfield, D. Theoretical nuances and practical old questions: The psychology of aging. *Canadian Psychologist*, 1972, *13*, 252–266.

Schonfield, D., & Robertson, E.A. Memory storage and aging. *Canadian Journal of Psychology*, 1966, *20*, 228–236.

Schonfield, D., & Stones, M.J. Remembering and aging. In J.F. Kihlstrom & F.J. Evans (Eds.), *Functional Disorders of Memory*. Hillsdale, N.J.: Lawrence Erlbaum Associates, 1979.

Schonfield, D., Trueman, V., & Kline, D. Recognition tests of dichotic listening and the age variable. *Journal of Gerontology*, 1972, *27*, 487–493.

Schonfield, D., & Wenger, L. Age limitation of perceptual span. *Nature*, 1975, *253*, 377–378.

Schwartz, D.W., & Karp, S.A. Field dependence in a geriatric population. *Perceptual and Motor Skills*, 1967, *24*, 495–504.

234   References

Sekuler, R., & Hutman, L.P. Spatial vision and aging: I. Contrast sensitivity. *Journal of Gerontology,* 1980, *35,* 692–699.

Sekuler, R., Hutman, L.P. & Owsley, C.J. Human aging and spatial vision. *Science,* 1980, *209,* 1255–1256.

Selzer, S.C., & Denney, N.W. Conservation abilities in middle-aged and elderly adults. *International Journal of Aging and Human Development,* 1980, *11,* 135–146.

Shagass, C., Amadeo, M., & Overton, D.A. Eye-tracking performance in psychiatric patients. *Biological Psychiatry,* 1974, *9,* 245–260.

Shakow, D., & Goldman, R. The effect of age on the Stanford-Binet vocabulary scores of adults. *Journal of Educational Psychology,* 1938, *31,* 241–256.

Shaps, L.P., & Nilsson, L.G. Encoding and retrieval operations in relation to age. *Developmental Psychology,* 1980, *16,* 636–643.

Sharpe, J.A., & Sylvester, T.O. Effect of aging on horizontal smooth pursuit. *Investigative Opthalomology and Visual Science,* 1978, *17,* 465–468.

Shepard, R., & Metzler, J. Mental rotation of three-dimensional objects. *Science,* 1971, *171,* 701–703.

Shiffrin, R.M., & Schneider, W. Controlled and automatic human information processing: II. Perceptual learning, automatic attending, and a general theory. *Psychological Review,* 1977, *84,* 127–190.

Silverman, I., & Reimanis, G. A test of two interpretations of age deficit in the ability to reverse an ambiguous figure. *Journal of Gerontology,* 1966, *21,* 89–92.

Simon, E. Depth and elaboration of processing in relation to age. *Journal of Experimental Psychology: Human Learning and Memory,* 1979, *5,* 115–124.

Simonson, E., Anderson, D., & Keiper, C. Effect of stimulus movement on critical flicker fusion in young and older men. *Journal of Gerontology,* 1967, *22,* 353–356.

Simonson, E., Enzer, N., & Blankstein, S.S. The influence of age on the fusion frequency of flicker. *Journal of Experimental Psychology,* 1941, *29,* 252–255.

Sivak, M., Olson, P.L., & Pastalan, L.A. Effect of driver's age on night-time legibility of highway signs. *Human Factors,* 1981, *23,* 59–64.

Sjostrom, K.P., & Pollack, R.H. The effect of simulated receptor aging on two types of visual illusions. *Psychonomic Science,* 1971, *23,* 147–148.

Slater, P. The association between age and score in the Progressive Matrices Test. *British Journal of Psychology Statistical Section,* 1948, *1,* 64–69.

Smith, A.D. Response interference with organized recall in the aged. *Developmental Psychology,* 1974, *10,* 867–870.

Smith, A.D. Aging and interference with memory. *Journal of Gerontology,* 1975, *30,* 319–325. (a)

Smith, A.D. Partial learning and recognition memory in the aged. *International Journal of Aging and Human Development,* 1975, *6,* 359–365. (b)

Smith, A.D. Aging and the total presentation time hypothesis. *Developmental Psychology,* 1976, *12,* 87–88.

Smith, A.D. Adult age differences in cued recall. *Developmental Psychology,* 1977, *13,* 326–331.

Smith, A.D. The interaction between age and list length in free recall. *Journal of Gerontology,* 1979, *34,* 375–380.

Smith, A.D. Age differences in encoding, storage and retrieval. In L.W. Poon, J.L. Fozard, L.S. Cermak, D. Arenberg, & L.W. Thompson (Eds.), *New Directions in Memory and Aging.* Hillsdale, N.J.: Lawrence Erlbaum Associates, 1980.

Smith, A.D., & Winograd, E. Age differences in recognizing faces. *Developmental Psychology*, 1978, *14*, 443–444.

Smith, M.E. Relation between word variety and mean letter length of words with chronological and mental ages. *Journal of General Psychology*, 1957, *56*, 27–43. (a)

Smith, M.E. The application of some measures of language behavior and tension to the letters written by a woman at each decade of her life from 49 to 89 years of age. *Journal of General Psychology*, 1957, *57*, 289–295. (b)

Somberg, B.L., & Salthouse, T.A. Divided-attention abilities in young and old adults. *Journal of Experimental Psychology: Human Perception and Performance*, in press.

Sorenson, H. Adult ages as a factor in learning. *Journal of Educational Psychology*, 1930, *21*, 451–459.

Sorenson, H. Mental ability over a wide range of adult ages. *Journal of Applied Psychology*, 1933, *17*, 729–741.

Sorenson, H. *Adult Abilities*, Minneapolis: University of Minnesota Press, 1938.

Speakman, D. The effect of age on the incidental relearning of stamp values. *Journal of Gerontology*, 1954, *9*, 162–167.

Spearman, C. *The Abilities of Man*. New York: MacMillan, 1927.

Sperling, G., & Melchner, M.J. Visual search, visual attention, and the attention-operating-characteristic. In J. Requin (Ed.), *Attention and Performance VII*. Hillsdale, N.J.: Lawrence Erlbaum Associates, 1978.

Squire, L.R. Remote memory as affected by aging. *Neuropsychologia*, 1974, *12*, 429–435.

Squire, L.R., & Fox, M.M. Assessment of remote memory: Validation of the television test by repeated testing during a 7-year period. *Behavior Research Methods and Instrumentation*, 1980, *12*, 583–586.

Sternberg, S. Memory scanning: Mental processes revealed by reaction time processes. *American Scientist*, 1969, *57*, 421–457.

Sternberg, S. Memory scanning: New findings and current controversies. *Quarterly Journal of Experimental Psychology*, 1975, *27*, 1–32.

Steven, D.M. Relation between dark adaptation and age. *Nature*, 1946, *157*, 376–377.

Storandt, M. Age, ability level, and method of administering and scoring the WAIS. *Journal of Gerontology*, 1977, *32*, 175–178.

Storandt, M., Grant, E.A., & Gordon, B.C. Remote memory as a function of age and sex. *Experimental Aging Research*, 1978, *4*, 365–375.

Storandt, M., & Hudson, W. Misuse of analysis of covariance in aging research and some partial solutions. *Experimental Aging Research*, 1975, *1*, 121–125.

Storck, P.A. & Looft, W.R. Qualitative analysis of vocabulary responses from persons aged six to sixty-six plus. *Journal of Educational Psychology*, 1973, *65*, 192–197.

Strother, C.R., Schaie, K.W., & Horst, P. The relationship between advanced age and mental abilities. *Journal of Abnormal and Social Psychology*, 1957, *55*, 166–170.

Suci, G.J., Davidoff, M.D., & Surwillo, W.W. Reaction time as a function of stimulus information and age. *Journal of Experimental Psychology*, 1960, *60*, 242–244.

Sward, K. Age and mental ability in superior men. *American Journal of Psychology*, 1945, *58*, 443–479.

Swensson, R.G. The elusive tradeoff: Speed vs. accuracy in visual discrimination tasks. *Perception and Psychophysics*, 1972, *12*, 16–32.

Szafran, J. Age differences in the rate of gain of information, signal detection strategy, and cardiovascular status among pilots. *Gerontologia*, 1966, *12*, 6–17.

Szafran, J. Psychophysiological studies of aging in pilots. In G.A. Talland (Ed.), *Human Aging and Behavior*. New York: Academic Press, 1968.

Talland, G.A. The effect of age on speed of simple manual skill. *Journal of Genetic Psychology*, 1962, *100*, 69–76.

Talland, G.A. Three estimates of the word span and their stability over the adult years. *Quarterly Journal of Experimental Psychology*, 1965, *17*, 301–307.

Talland, G.A. Age and the immediate memory span. *Gerontologist*, 1967, *7*, 4–9.

Talland, G.A. Age and the span of immediate recall. In G.A. Talland (Ed.), *Human Aging and Behavior*. New York: Academic Press, 1968.

Taub, H.A. Visual short-term memory as a function of age, rate of presentation, and schedule of presentation. *Journal of Gerontology*, 1966, *21*, 388–391.

Taub, H.A. Paired-associates learning as a function of age, rate and instructions. *Journal of Genetic Psychology*, 1967, *111*, 41–46.

Taub, H.A. Age differences in memory as a function of rate of presentation, order of report, and stimulus organization. *Journal of Gerontology*, 1968, *23*, 159–164.

Taub, H.A. A comparison of young adult and old groups on various digit span tasks. *Developmental Psychology*, 1972, *6*, 60–65.

Taub, H.A. Memory span, practice, and aging. *Journal of Gerontology*, 1973, *28*, 335–338.

Taub, H.A. Coding for short-term memory as a function of age. *Journal of Genetic Psychology*, 1974, *125*, 309–314.

Taub, H.A. Mode of presentation, age, and short-term memory. *Journal of Gerontology*, 1975, *30*, 56–59.

Taub, H.A. Method of presentation of meaningful prose to young and old adults. *Experimental Aging Research*, 1976, *2*, 469–474.

Taub, H.A., & Kline, G.E. Modality effects and memory in the aged. *Educational Gerontology*, 1976, *1*, 53–60.

Taub, H.A., & Long, M.K. The effects of practice on short-term memory of young and old subjects. *Journal of Gerontology*, 1972, *27*, 494–499.

Taylor, M.M., Lindsay, P.H., & Forbes, S.M. Quantification of shared capacity processing in auditory and visual discrimination. In A.F. Sanders (Ed.), *Attention and Performance, I*. Amsterdam: North-Holland, 1967.

Tesch, S., Whitbourne, S.K., & Nehrke, M.F. Cognitive egocentrism in institutionalized adult males. *Journal of Gerontology*, 1978, *33*, 546–552.

Thomas, E.A.C. The selectivity of preparation. *Psychological Review*, 1974, *81*, 442–464.

Thomas, J.C., Fozard, J.L., & Waugh, N.C. Age-related differences in naming latency. *American Journal of Psychology*, 1977, *90*, 499–509.

Thomas, J.M., & Charles, D.C. Effects of age and stimulus size on perception. *Journal of Gerontology*, 1964, *19*, 447–450.

Thorndike, E.L., Bregman, E.O., Tilton, J.W., & Woodyard, E. *Adult Learning*. New York: MacMillan, 1928.

Thorndike, E.L., & Gallup, G.H. Verbal intelligence of the American adult. *Journal of General Psychology*, 1944, *30*, 75–85.

Till, R.E. Age-related differences in binocular backward masking with visual noise. *Journal of Gerontology*, 1978, *33*, 702–710.

Till, R.E., & Franklin, L.D. On the locus of age differences in visual information processing. *Journal of Gerontology*, 1981, *36*, 200–210.

Till, R.E., & Walsh, D.A. Encoding and retreival factors in adult memory for implicational sentences. *Journal of Verbal Learning and Verbal Behavior*, 1980, *19*, 1–16.

Traxler, A.J. Retroactive and proactive inhibition in young and elderly adults using an unpaced modified free-recall test. *Psychological Reports*, 1973, *32*, 215–222.

Treat, N.J., Poon, L.W., & Fozard, J.L. Age, imagery, and practice in paired-associated learning. *Experimental Aging Research*, 1981, *7*, 337–342.

Treat, N.J., Poon, L.W., Fozard, J.L., & Popkin, S.J. Toward applying cognitive skill training to memory problems. *Experimental Aging Research*, 1978, *4*, 305–319.

Treat, N.J., & Reese, H.W. Age, pacing and imagery in paired-associate learning. *Developmental Psychology*, 1976, *12*, 119–124.

Trembly, D., & O'Connor, J. Growth and decline of natural and acquired intellectual characteristics. *Journal of Gerontology*, 1966, *21*, 9–12.

Tresselt, M.E., & Mayzner, M.S. The Kent-Rosanoff Word Association: Word association norms as a function of age. *Psychonomic Science*, 1964, *1*, 65–66.

Tuddenham, R.D. Soldier intelligence in World Wars I and II. *American Psychologist*, 1948, *3*, 54–56.

Tuddenham, R.D., Blumenkrantz, J., & Wilkin, W.R. Age changes on AGCT: A longitudinal study of average adults. *Journal of Consulting and Clinical Psychology*, 1968, *32*, 659–663.

Tulving, E. Episodic and semantic memory. In E. Tulving & W. Donaldson (Eds.), *Organization of Memory*. New York: Academic Press, 1972.

Tulving, E., & Colotla, V. Free recall of trilingual lists. *Cognitive Psychology*, 1970, *1*, 86–98.

Tulving, E., & Patterson, R.D. Functional units and retrieval processes in free recall. *Journal of Experimental Psychology*, 1968, *77*, 239–248.

Tulving, E., & Thomson, D.M. Encoding specificity and retrieval processes in episodic memory. *Psychological Review*, 1973, *80*, 352–373.

Verhage, F. Intelligence and age in a Dutch sample. *Human Development*, 1965, *8*, 238–245.

Verrillo, R.T. Absolute estimation of line length in three age groups. *Journal of Gerontology*, 1981, *36*, 625–627.

Verville, E., & Cameron, N. Age and sex differences in the perception of incomplete pictures by adults. *Journal of Genetic Psychology*, 1946, *68*, 149–157.

Vincent, D.F. The linear relationship between age and score of adults in intelligence tests. *Occupational Psychology*, 1952, *26*, 243–249.

Waddell, K.J., & Rogoff, B. Effect of contextual organization on spatial memory of middle-aged and older women. *Developmental Psychology*, 1981, *17*, 878–885.

Walker, J.F. The job performance of federal mail sorters by age. *Monthly Labor Review*, 1964, *87*, 296–300.

Wallace, J.G. Some studies of perception in relation to age. *British Journal of Psychology*, 1956, *47*, 283–297.

Walsh, D.A. Age differences in learning and memory. In D.S. Woodruff & J.E. Birren (Eds.), *Aging: Scientific Perspectives and Social Issues*. New York: Van Nostrand, 1975.

Walsh, D.A. Age differences in central perceptual processing: A dichoptic masking investigation. *Journal of Gerontology*, 1976, *31*, 178–185.

Walsh, D.A., & Baldwin, M. Age differences in integrated semantic memory. *Developmental Psychology*, 1977, *13*, 509–514.

Walsh, D.A., Baldwin, M., & Finkle, T.J. Age differences in integrated semantic memory for abstract sentences. *Experimental Aging Research,* 1980, *6,* 431–444.

Walsh, D.A., & Prasse, M.J. Iconic memory and attentional processes in the aged. In L.W. Poon, J.L. Fozard, L.S. Cermak, D. Arenberg, & L.W. Thompson (Eds.), *New Directions in Memory and Aging.* Hillsdale, N.J.: Lawrence Erlbaum Associates, 1980.

Walsh, D.A., & Thompson, L.W. Age differences in visual sensory memory. *Journal of Gerontology,* 1978, *33,* 383–387.

Walsh, D.A., Till, R.E., & Williams, M.V. Age differences in peripheral perceptual processing: A monoptic backward masking investigation. *Journal of Experimental Psychology: Human Perception and Performance,* 1978, *4,* 232–243.

Walsh, D.A., Williams, M.V., & Hertzog, C.K. Age-related differences in two stages of central perceptual processes: The effects of short-duration targets and criterion differences. *Journal of Gerontology,* 1979, *34,* 234–241.

Wapner, S., Werner, H., & Comalli, P.E. Perception of part-whole relationships in middle and old age. *Journal of Gerontology,* 1960, *15,* 412–418.

Warren, L.R., & Mitchell, S.A. Age differences in judging the frequency of events. *Developmental Psychology,* 1980, *16,* 116–120.

Warren, R.E. Stimulus encoding and memory. *Journal of Experimental Psychology,* 1972, *94,* 90–100.

Warrington, E.K., & Sanders, H.I. The fate of old memories. *Quarterly Journal of Experimental Psychology,* 1971, *23,* 432–442.

Watkins, M.J. Concept and measurement of primary memory. *Psychological Bulletin,* 1974, *81,* 695–711.

Waugh, N.C., & Barr, R.A. Memory and mental tempo. In L.W. Poon, J.L. Fozard, L.S. Cermak, D. Arenberg, & L.W. Thompson (Eds.), *New Directions in Memory and Aging.* Hillsdale, N.J.: Lawrence Erlbaum Associates, 1980.

Wechsler, D. *Measurement of Adult Intelligence.* Baltimore: The Williams & Wilkins Co., 1939.

Wechsler, D. *Measurement of Adult Intelligence,* 4th Ed., Baltimore, MD.: The Williams & Wilkins Co., 1958.

Weiner, M. Organization of mental abilities from ages 14 to 54. *Educational and Psychological Measurement,* 1964, *24,* 573–587.

Weisenburg, T., Roe, A., & McBride, K.E. *Adult Intelligence.* New York: The Commonwealth Fund, 1936.

Welford, A.T. Methodological problems in the study of changes in human performance with age. In G.E.W. Wolstenholme & C.M. O'Connor (Eds.), *Ciba Foundation Colloquia on Ageing (Vol. 3).* London: Churchill, 1957.

Welford, A.T. *Ageing and Human Skill.* London: Oxford University Press, 1958.

Welford, A.T. Changes in the speed of performance with age and their industrial significance. *Ergonomics,* 1962, *5,* 139–145.

Welford, A.T. Motor performance. In J.E. Birren & K.W. Schaie (Eds.), *Handbook of the Psychology of Aging.* New York: Van Nostrand Reinhold, 1977.

Welsandt, R.F., Zupnick, J.J., & Meyer, P.A. Age effects in backward visual masking (Crawford Paradigm). *Journal of Experimental Child Psychology,* 1973, *15,* 454–461.

Weston, H.C. The effect of age and illumination upon visual performance with close sights. *British Journal of Opthalomology,* 1948, *32,* 645–653.

Westworth-Rohr, I., Mackintosh, R.M., & Fialkoff, B.S. The relationship of Hooper VOT score to sex, education, intelligence, and age. *Journal of Clinical Psychology,* 1974, *30,* 73–75.

Wetherwick, N.E. Changing an established concept: A comparison of the ability of young, middle-aged, and old subjects. *Gerontologia,* 1965, *11,* 82–95.

Whitbourne, S.K., & Slevin, A.G. Imagery and sentence retention in elderly and young adults. *Journal of Genetic Psychology,* 1978, *133,* 287–298.

Whiteman, M., & Jastak, J. Absolute scaling of tests for a state-wide sample. *Educational and Psychological Measurement,* 1957, *17,* 338–346.

Wickelgren, W.K. Age and storage dynamics in continuous recognition memory. *Developmental Psychology,* 1975, *11,* 165–169.

Wickens, D.D. Characteristics of word encoding. In A.W. Melton & E. Martin (Eds.), *Coding Processes in Human Memory.* Washington, D.C.: Winston & Sons, 1972.

Wiersma, W., & Klausmeier, H.J. The effect of age upon speed of concept attainment. *Journal of Gerontology,* 1965, *20,* 398–400.

Williams, M. The effect of past experience on mental performance in the elderly. *British Journal of Medical Psychology,* 1960, *33,* 215–221.

Willis, S.L., & Baltes, P.B. Intelligence in adulthood and aging: Contemporary issues. In L.W. Poon (Ed.), *Aging in the 1980's.* Washington, D.C.: American Psychological Association, 1980.

Willoughby, R.R. Family similarities in mental test abilities (with a note on the growth and decline of these abilities). *Genetic Psychology Monographs,* 1927, *2,* 235–277.

Willoughby, R.R. Incidental learning. *Journal of Educational Psychology,* 1929, *20,* 671–682.

Wilson, J.R., DeFries, J.G., McClearn, G.E., Vandenberg, S.G., Johnson, R.C., & Rashad, M.N. Cognitive abilities: Use of family data as a control to assess sex and age differences in two ethnic groups. *International Journal of Aging and Human Development,* 1975, *6,* 261–276.

Wilson, T.R. Flicker fusion frequency, age, and intelligence. *Gerontologia,* 1963, *7,* 200–208.

Wimer, R.E. Age differences in incidental and intentional learning. *Journal of Gerontology,* 1960, *15,* 79–82. (a)

Wimer, R.E. A supplementary report on age differences in retention over a twenty-four hour period. *Journal of Gerontology,* 1960, *15,* 417–418. (b)

Wimer, R.E., & Wigdor, B.T. Age differences in retention of learning. *Journal of Gerontology,* 1958, *13,* 291–295.

Winn, F.J., Elias, J.W., & Marshall, P.H. Meaningfulness and interference as factors in paired-associate learning with the aged. *Educational Gerontology,* 1976, *1,* 297–306.

Winograd, E., & Simon, E.W. Visual memory and imagery in the aged. In L.W. Poon, J.L. Fozard, L.S. Cermak, D. Arenberg, & L.W. Thompson (Eds.), *New Directions in Memory and Aging.* Hillsdale, N.J.: Lawrence Erlbaum Associates, 1980.

Winograd, E., Smith, A.D., & Simon, E.W. Aging and the picture superiority effect in recall. *Journal of Gerontology,* 1982, *37,* 70–75.

Witte, K.L., & Freund, J.S. Paired-associate learning in young and old adults as related to stimulus concreteness and presentation method. *Journal of Gerontology,* 1976, *31,* 186–192.

Wittels, I. Age and stimulus meaningfulness in paired-associate learning. *Journal of Gerontology,* 1972, *27,* 372–375.

Wohlwill, J.F. Methodology and research strategy in the study of developmental change. In L.R. Goulet & P.B. Baltes (Eds.), *Life-Span Developmental Psychology: Research and Theory.* New York: Academic Press, 1970.

Wolf, E. Glare and age. *A.M.A. Archives in Opthalomology,* 1960, *64,* 502–514.

Wolf, E. Studies on the shrinkage of the visual field with age. *Highway Research Record,* 1967, *167,* 1–7.

Wright, L.L., & Elias, J.W. Age differences in the effects of perceptual noise. *Journal of Gerontology,* 1979, *34,* 704–708.

Wright, R.E. Aging, divided attention, and processing capacity. *Journal of Gerontology,* 1981, *36,* 605–614.

Wright, R.E. Adult age similarities in free-recall output order and strategies. *Journal of Gerontology,* 1982, *37,* 76–79.

Yerkes, R.M. Psychological examining in the United States Army. *Memoirs of the National Academy of Sciences,* 1921, *15,* 1–877.

Young, M.L. Problem-solving performance in two age groups. *Journal of Gerontology,* 1966, *21,* 505–509.

Zaretsky, H., & Halberstam, J. Effects of aging, brain damage, and associative strength on paired-associate learning and relearning. *Journal of Genetic Psychology,* 1968, *112,* 149–163.

Zarit, S.H., Cole, K.D., & Guider, R.L. Memory training strategies and subjective complaints of memory in the aged. *Gerontologist,* 1981, *21,* 158–164.

Zelinski, E.M., Gilewski, M.J., & Thompson, L.W. Do laboratory tasks relate to self-assessment of memory ability in the young and old? In L.W. Poon, J.L. Fozard, L.S. Cermak, D. Arenberg, & L.W. Thompson (Eds.), *New Directions in Memory and Aging.* Hillsdale, N.J.: Lawrence Erlbaum Associates, 1980.

Zelinski, E.M., Walsh, D.A., & Thompson, L.W. Orienting task effects on EDR and free recall in three age groups. *Journal of Gerontology,* 1978, *33,* 239–245.

Author Index

Note: Entries in italics refer to References

Subject Index